ABC of
Medically Unexplained Symptoms

ABC series

An outstanding collection of resources for everyone in primary care

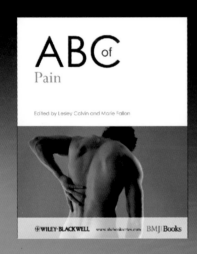

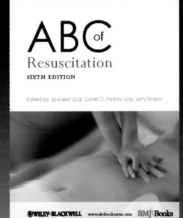

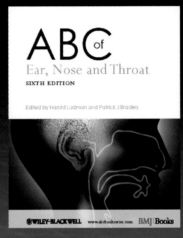

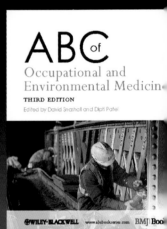

The *ABC* series contains a wealth of indispensable resources for GPs, GP registrars, junior doctors, doctors in training and all those in primary care

▶ **Highly illustrated, informative and a practical source of knowledge**

▶ **An easy-to-use resource, covering the symptoms, investigations, treatment and management of conditions presenting in day-to-day practice and patient support**

▶ **Full colour photographs and illustrations aid diagnosis and patient understanding of a condition**

For more information on all books in the *ABC* series, including links to further information, references and links to the latest official guidelines, please visit:

www.abcbookseries.com

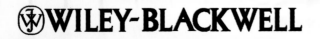

⟨W⟩ WILEY-BLACKWELL　　　　　　BMJ|Book

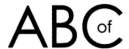

ABC of

Medically Unexplained Symptoms

EDITED BY

Christopher Burton

Senior Lecturer in Primary Care
University of Aberdeen, UK

WILEY-BLACKWELL

A John Wiley & Sons, Ltd., Publication

BMJ|Books

Library of Congress Cataloging-in-Publication Data

ABC of medically unexplained symptoms / edited by Chris Burton.

p. ; cm.

Includes bibliographical references and index.

ISBN 978-1-119-96725-5 (pbk.)

I. Burton, Chris, 1958-

[DNLM: 1. Signs and Symptoms. 2. Diagnosis. 3. Primary Health Care–methods. WB 143]

616.07′5–dc23

2012032698

A catalogue record for this book is available from the British Library.

Wiley also publishes its books in a variety of electronic formats. Some content that appears in print may not be available in electronic books.

Cover image: Sickle cell disease clinic C0105521 Copyright © 2011 LIFE IN VIEW/SCIENCE PHOTO LIBRARY
Cover design by: Meaden Creative

Set in 9.25/12 Minion by Laserwords Private Limited, Chennai, India
Printed and bound in Malaysia by Vivar Printing Sdn Bhd

1 2013

Contents

Contributors

Chris Burton
Senior Lecturer in Primary Care,
University of Aberdeen, Aberdeen, UK

Camille Busby-Earle
Consultant Gynaecologist, Simpson Centre for Reproductive Health,
Royal Infirmary of Edinburgh, Edinburgh, UK

Alan Carson
Senior Lecturer in Psychiatry, Robert Fergusson Unit,
University of Edinburgh, Edinburgh, UK

Nur Amalina Che Bakri
MRC Centre for Reproductive Health, University of Edinburgh,
Edinburgh, UK

Avril F. Danczak
Primary Care Medical Educator, Central and South Manchester Speciality
Training Programme for General Practice, North Western Deanery and
Principal, The Alexandra Practice, Manchester, UK

Vincent Deary
Senior Lecturer in Psychology, Department of Psychology,
University of Northumbria, Newcastle, UK

Christopher Dowrick
Professor of Primary Care, Department of Mental and Behavioural Health
Sciences, University of Liverpool, Liverpool, UK

Andrew W. Horne
Senior Lecturer and Consultant Gynaecologist, MRC Centre for
Reproductive Health, University of Edinburgh, Edinburgh, UK

David P. Kernick
General Practitioner, St Thomas Medical Group, Exeter, UK

Christian Mallen
Professor of General Practice, Arthritis Research UK Primary Care Centre,
Keele University, Keele, UK

John McBeth
Reader in Chronic Pain Epidemiology, Arthritis Research UK Primary Care
Centre, Keele University, Keele, UK

Barbara Nicholl
Research Associate, Arthritis Research UK Primary Care Centre,
Keele University, Keele, UK

Alexandra Rolfe
Academic Clinical Fellow in General Practice, Centre for Population Health
Sciences, University of Edinburgh, Edinburgh, UK

Robby Steel
Consultant Psychiatrist, Department of Psychological Medicine, Royal
Infirmary of Edinburgh, Edinburgh, UK

Jon Stone
Consultant Neurologist and Honorary Senior Lecturer in Neurology,
Department of Clinical Neurosciences, Western General Hospital,
Edinburgh, UK

Henriëtte E. van der Horst
Professor, Head of General Practice Department. VU Medical Centre,
Amsterdam, The Netherlands

Alison J. Wearden
Professor of Health Psychology, School of Psychological Sciences,
Astley Ainslie Hospital & University of Manchester, Manchester, UK

Killian A. Welch
Honorary Clinical Senior Lecturer, Robert Fergusson Unit,
University of Edinburgh, Edinburgh, UK

David Weller
Professor of General Practice, Centre for Population Health Sciences,
University of Edinburgh, Edinburgh, UK

Acknowledgements

In compiling this book I have drawn on the insights not only of the chapter authors, but on many other people over a long time. Some of these have been clinical colleagues, particularly at Sanquhar Health Centre where I have been privileged to work for 26 years. Some have been fellow academics who have supported and guided my research career. Most, however, have been patients who have encouraged me to think in terms of symptoms as experiences to be understood and dealt with in a range of ways. This book would not have been possible without them.

CHAPTER 1

Introduction

Chris Burton

University of Aberdeen, Aberdeen, UK

> **OVERVIEW**
>
> - Medically unexplained symptoms (MUS) are characterised by disturbances of function – including physiological, neurological and cognitive processes
> - Using what is currently known about disturbed function, it is possible to develop coherent and plausible models of conditions in order to explain what is going on to patients
> - Sharing explanations and understanding concerns allows the doctor and patient to work together. Describing symptoms as disorders of function is an acceptable way of doing this

Aim

This book aims to help general practitioners (GPs) and other generalists to understand and treat conditions associated with symptoms that appear not to be caused by physical disease. This lack of explanation due to visible pathology means they are often called medically unexplained symptoms (MUS). This book takes the view that MUS are disorders of function, rather than structure, and so the book will refer to them as functional symptoms. Although we do not fully understand the nature of the disturbed function, research is making this clearer and several mechanisms, including physiological, neurological and cognitive processes play a part in symptoms. This book also takes the view that by using what is currently known about functional symptoms, it is possible to develop coherent and plausible models to explain what is going on. This book aims to help doctors explain the medically unexplained – both to themselves and to their patients.

Symptoms that appear not to be caused by physical disease are a challenge to doctors and patients. Both have to simultaneously consider the possibility of serious illness (either physical or mental) while seeking to contain and reduce the symptoms and the threat they represent. This is not easy. In order to deal with MUS, and the patients who present with them, doctors need to apply a range of clinical skills: from empathic history taking and

focused examination, through careful assessment of probabilities, to communication, explanation and – sometimes – support. This book assumes you already have those skills to some extent; it aims to show ways of using, and developing, them in order to deal with these common problems.

An approach to MUS

The *ABC of Medically Unexplained Symptoms* is not a book about the somatisation of mental distress from a psychoanalytic perspective. It does not take the view that unexplained symptoms are a way of communicating need in people who cannot otherwise do so. Rather it takes a mechanistic view of symptoms as the result of interacting processes – some physiological, some neuropsychological – that lead to persistent unpleasant feelings and distress. This approach is similar to that used in pain medicine, with which it has much in common; indeed many unexplained symptoms and syndromes include pain.

This introductory chapter addresses three questions: what do we mean by medically unexplained symptoms; what causes medically unexplained symptoms; and what should we call medically unexplained symptoms?

What do we mean by medically unexplained symptoms?

The simple answer to this question is 'physical symptoms that cannot be explained by disease', but it has several problems. First, this book is written largely from a primary care perspective and although it may be that every possible disease has been ruled out in tertiary care, this is not often the case in primary care. Furthermore, not all 'diseases' have consistent pathology – migraine is an excellent example of a syndrome that we have kept on the 'explained' side of the dividing line between explained and medically unexplained symptoms but where the problem is one of disturbed function rather than structure. Even persistent back pain, which initially seems an obvious 'explained' symptom, shows almost no correlation between symptom severity and structural abnormality.

Instead of this simple 'absence of disease' answer, it can be helpful to think of three different meanings: symptoms with low probability of disease; functional somatic syndromes; and experiencing multiple physical symptoms. This book will use

---

ABC of Medically Unexplained Symptoms, First Edition.
Edited by Christopher Burton.
© 2013 John Wiley & Sons, Ltd. Published 2013 by John Wiley & Sons, Ltd.

the adjective 'functional' in relation to symptoms or syndromes (i.e. MUS) to mean simply that we can best understand them in terms of disturbed function without altered structure. In general it will use the term 'organic' to refer to conditions associated with pathological change.

Symptoms with low probability of disease

This term has recently been introduced in an attempt to capture the uncertainty that is inherent in this field. Around 10% of patients in primary care with persistent so-called MUS eventually turn out to have an alternative diagnosis. The proportion is rather lower in some forms of secondary care but nonetheless all doctors will have seen a patient whom they originally thought had a functional symptom but turned out to have a disease. We believe that the concept of symptoms with low probability of disease is useful though, as it can be applied to a patient with positive pointers to a functional disorder and with no red flags for serious illness to indicate a 'working diagnosis'. Chapters 3 and 4 describe the recognition of physical illness and emotional disorders in patients with MUS.

Functional somatic syndromes

The common functional physical symptoms – fatigue, headache, light-headedness, headache, palpitations, chest pain, nausea, bloating, abdominal pain, musculoskeletal pain and weakness often occur together. Some of these clusters – particularly when they present to a given clinical specialty – are commonly grouped together as a syndrome. So gastroenterology has the irritable bowel syndrome (IBS), rheumatology has chronic widespread pain and fibromyalgia, and gynaecologists have chronic pelvic pain. As Figure 1.1 shows, and as described further in Chapter 2, all these symptoms overlap; to the extent that some experts argue that all the syndromes represent facets of a single disorder.

In practical terms, however, the syndrome labels are here to stay and they often represent useful diagnostic labels or categories. The common syndromes are covered in this book, and when we use the term 'MUS', it includes these defined syndromes as well as less clearly categorised symptoms.

Experiencing multiple physical symptoms

As Chapter 2 describes, everyone has some functional symptoms at some point in their life. What matters is that some patients have multiple physical symptoms that cause distress and that have an impact in terms of restricting behaviour or seeking medical attention. This triad of multiple symptoms, distress and impact has received various names including somatisation (but it then gets confused with the psychoanalytic concept) and most recently a proposed new term 'bodily distress disorder'. At the moment there is no widely acceptable name for this phenomenon, but the triad of multiple symptoms (Box 1.1), distress and impact seems to describe an important group of patients well.

> Box 1.1 **The triad of experiencing multiple symptoms**
>
> - Experiencing multiple symptoms
> - Distress because of symptoms
> - Impact on activities or healthcare seeking because of symptoms

What causes MUS?

The simple answer is 'we don,'t know' – because otherwise they wouldn't be medically unexplained symptoms. But actually we know quite a bit about the factors that predispose patients to MUS, the mechanisms that give rise to symptoms; the cognitive processes by which they are appraised and the processes that perpetuate them.

Predisposing factors

If you have the good fortune to have been born with the right genes, brought up in an emotionally secure family, protected from

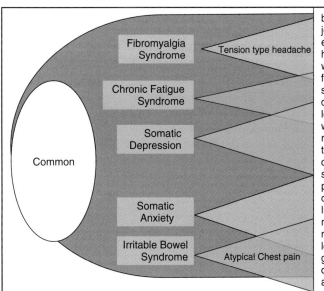

Figure 1.1 Overlap of medically unexplained symptoms.

poverty, illness and abuse, and have a fulfilling role in life then your chances of problems with MUS (and most other conditions) are reduced. However for most people it is difficult to argue that one factor is more important than another. Depression and anxiety undoubtedly predispose to future MUS, and conversely MUS predispose to future depression and anxiety.

Biological mechanisms

Given that there is no obvious disorder of structure, it is reasonable – and acceptable – to talk of MUS as disorders of function and you will find this sort of language in several of the chapters. As well as more obvious changes of function such as gut motility or heart rate, subtle changes in autonomic function are common in patients with MUS. Some form of hypothalamic–pituitary axis dysfunction appears to be present in many patients with fatigue and chronic pain and there is mounting evidence for the effect of stress on immune regulation.

Central sensitisation to pain is an increasingly recognised and understood process in all forms of chronic pain (whether 'explained' or not). It is characterised by heightened perception of, and distress from, a range of sensory inputs and includes the two components hyperalgesia (heightened perception of painful stimuli) and allodynia (pain arising from non-painful stimuli) illustrated in Figure 1.2. Neuroimaging is beginning to highlight characteristic areas of under- and overactivity as symptoms are processed in the brain. This is an active field of research and it seems inevitable that new physical mechanisms will be uncovered with time.

Symptom awareness and appraisal

It is important to recognise that symptoms feel the same to the patient, whether they are 'explained' or 'medically unexplained'. This is important to convey to patients who sometimes think that if no physical cause can be found then the doctor thinks they are imagining it – and that, somehow, functional symptoms would feel different.

The same centres in the brain are activated regardless of the origin of pain and detailed studies of the experience of symptoms show that distress from and response to symptoms follow similar patterns, regardless of cause. The experience of symptoms is a complex phenomenon: incoming stimuli to the brain pass through a series of stages before they reach awareness: these are outlined in Box 1.2.

Box 1.2 **Stages in the response to an incoming unpleasant stimulus**

1 *Reflex expression of emotion*: for example fear or disgust. This triggering is involuntary and emotion itself causes its own actions.
2 *Checking against memory*: by the time a person becomes aware of a symptom, they are already experiencing the emotional response and have compared it *with* other experiences.
3 *Deciding what to do*: this stage of symptom appraisal means that once aware of something we already have an idea *of* what to do. Often it is just nothing, but some patients have particular responses, with perfectly rational reasons.

If you think this sounds a bit improbable, consider the account of anxious people who have noticed extrasystoles when resting. The awareness of even a single extra heartbeat already comes with a sense of anxiety and 'oh no, not again, I need to get out of here'.

Perpetuating factors

A common way of making sense of functional symptoms is to consider perpetuating cycles. Figure 1.3 shows two examples: in each case the cycle is triggered by a short-lived incident (for instance a virus infection in the fatigue cycle) but then may become self-perpetuating. The second example is based on the cognitive model of panic but is applicable to other symptoms. It includes an extra loop of increased awareness that means that

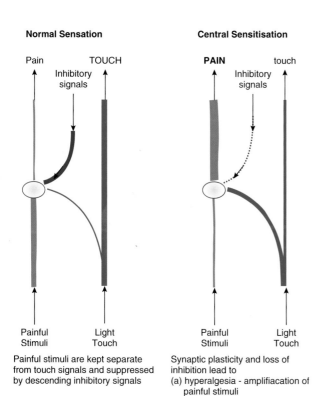

Normal Sensation

Painful stimuli are kept separate from touch signals and suppressed by descending inhibitory signals

Central Sensitisation

Synaptic plasticity and loss of inhibition lead to
(a) hyperalgesia - amplifiacation of painful stimuli
(b) allodynia - pain arising from non-painful stimuli

Figure 1.2 Sensory pathways in normal sensation and central sensitisation.

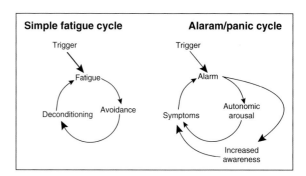

Figure 1.3 Cycles of perpetuating processes.

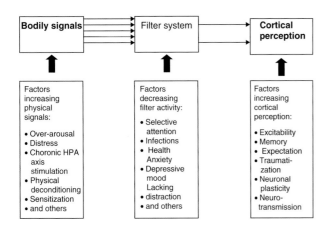

Figure 1.4 A filter model for Medically unexplained symptoms. HPA, hypothalamic–pituitary–adrenal. Reprinted from Rief W and Broadbent E. Explaining medically unexplained symptoms – models and mechanisms. *Clinical Psychology Review* **27** (2007) 821–841. Copyright © 2007, with permission from Elsevier.

minor autonomic changes, which might otherwise go unnoticed, are perceived and thus regarded as abnormal and hence processed as symptoms, generating further alarm. This model is particularly applicable to a range of autonomic symptoms such as palpitations or lightheadedness.

An integrated model

Figure 1.4 shows a model that integrates predisposing factors, causal mechanisms, symptom appraisal and perpetuating factors. It uses the idea of filters in a way that is analogous to the gate theory of pain. This model is a coherent attempt to bring together multiple factors and also has the advantage that problems can be explained as failure of the filters (or 'barriers'). Many patients find 'your pain (or symptom) barriers aren't working' to be less judgemental than 'your nerves have become more sensitive'. Repairing these barriers then becomes a useful objective for therapeutic work.

What should we call MUS?

The simple answer to this is 'whatever you and your patient find useful'. There are no good terms here, just less bad ones. In the rankings of things not to say to patients, 'All in the mind' and 'psychosomatic' are the worst. They have a Number Needed to Offend of only 2 or 3!

The symptom syndromes can be a valuable way of legitimising symptoms for patients, particularly when the symptoms have been present for several months. When symptoms are more recent, it is still usually acceptable to talk about functional symptoms – as long as you indicate that you are using that term because of features of disturbed bodily function.

How to use this book

The chapters of this book should be considered as being in three sections. The first (Chapters 1–6) represents an introduction and overview, with chapters about the epidemiology and impact of MUS, suspecting physical and mental illness and a consideration of some of the specific problems for doctors that MUS brings. It ends with a chapter outlining a set of principles for the management of patients with MUS. This section is designed to be read through, reflectively. Its contents are at the heart of clinical practice and comprise appropriate material for self-directed learning in terms of appraisal and revalidation.

The second part of the book (Chapters 7–13) covers commonly occurring MUS in a range of specialties. These are designed to be dipped into, on an as-needed basis.

The final section (Chapters 14–18) considers treatment from a range of perspectives. Like the first section of the book, it is designed to be read through and digested. It contains tips for generalists as well as descriptions of the sort of things specialists will do when treating the generalist's patients.

You might wish to use your learning from this book as part of a personal development plan towards revalidation. In order to help with this, and to increase its impact, the Appendix suggests points for reflection and audit based on each chapter that represent a starting point for further thought.

This book cannot tell you everything you might want to know about MUS, but hopefully it combines an overall approach that is practical and useful, with sufficient information about specific conditions to help you manage them well.

Further reading

Burton C. Beyond somatisation: a review of the understanding and management of medically unexplained physical symptoms (MUPS). *Br J GenPract* 2003;**53**:233–241.

Henningsen P, Jakobsen T, Schiltenwolf M, Weiss MG. Somatization revisited: diagnosis and perceived causes of common mental disorders. *J Nerv Ment Dis* 2005;**193**:85–92.

Henningsen P, Zipfel S, Herzog W. Management of functional somatic syndromes. *Lancet* 2007;**369**:946–55.

Rief W, Broadbent E. Explaining medically unexplained symptoms – models and mechanisms. *Clin Psychol Rev* 2007;**27**:821–41.

Sharpe M, Mayou R, Walker J. Bodily symptoms: new approaches to classification. *J Psychosom Res* 2006;**60**:353–6.

CHAPTER 2

Epidemiology and Impact in Primary and Secondary Care

Alexandra Rolfe[1] and Chris Burton[2]

[1]Centre for Population Health Sciences, University of Edinburgh, Edinburgh, UK
[2]University of Aberdeen, Aberdeen, UK

OVERVIEW

- Medically unexplained symptoms (MUS) are common in all fields of medicine
- Many patients have only occasional or mild MUS, but some have either persistent, recurring or changing symptoms
- In addition to the distress they cause to patients, MUS are a public health issue due to their prevalence and associated resource cost

---

Epidemiology

Symptoms that cannot be adequately explained by disease are common in almost all fields of medicine. The term MUS includes symptoms that are part of a recognised syndrome (such as IBS or fibromyalgia) as well as those symptoms that are not, for instance intermittent palpitations or fatigue of less than 6 months duration.

The prevalence of MUS can be considered at three levels: the general population, GP consulters and patients referred from primary to secondary care.

Population prevalence

Most people will have at least one MUS that is sufficiently severe for them to seek medical advice at some point in their life. In that respect, an occasional symptom not due to disease can be regarded as normal. Between 10 and 20% of adults will have experienced several MUS (more than 4 for men or 6 for women, from a list of 30) over their life course. These epidemiological criteria are sometimes referred to as somatoform disorder or abridged somatisation.

Only around 0.2% of adults have the most severe form of MUS known as somatisation disorder, which is characterised by experiencing, and seeking treatment for, many MUS and starting before the age of 30.

GP consultation prevalence

Estimates of the proportion of patients consulting a GP with MUS vary. A commonly quoted figure is 15%, which is roughly equivalent to one patient per hour of clinic time based on 10 min appointments. Of course, some days it will be less, some days it will feel like much more!

More important than the prevalence of a single MUS in GP clinics is the proportion of patients who repeatedly attend with MUS. This seems to be about 2% of the practice population – and is similar whether one looks at patients who attend repeatedly with MUS over a year or those who are referred to specialists with MUS at least twice over a period of 5 years. Given that these people are relatively frequent consulters, they are likely to account for 4–6% of consultations or one to two patients per day.

Referral prevalence

MUS are common among patients referred to specialists. Table 2.1 shows the proportion of patients referred to six specialties who were deemed by the specialist to have no organic disease. Sometimes referral for MUS is necessary in order to make a diagnosis (for instance see Chapter 13) but in other cases there may be a very low probability of disease and it seems likely that GPs refer some patients for reassurance, either of the patient or themselves.

Prevalence and overlap of syndromes

Many patients with MUS meet criteria for a syndrome such as IBS or fibromyalgia. Population surveys demonstrate that these are all fairly common, although most patients with them do not consult their GP. Although the use of syndrome labels encourages us to think about them as discrete entities, it is clear that there

Table 2.1 Prevalence of medically unexplained symptoms in new referrals to different specialities.

Speciality	Prevalence (%)
Cardiology	53
Gastroenterology	58
Gynaecology	66
Neurology	62
Respiratory	41
Rheumatology	45

ABC of Medically Unexplained Symptoms, First Edition.
Edited by Christopher Burton.
© 2013 John Wiley & Sons, Ltd. Published 2013 by John Wiley & Sons, Ltd.

Table 2.2 Proportion of patients with one functional syndrome who also had another, among hospital outpatient attenders.

Patients with	n	Proportion (%) who also had					
		TTH	NCCP	FM	IBS	CFS	CPP
Tension-type headache	99		24	34	28	22	18
Non-cardiac chest pain	96	25		21	16	12	9
Fibromyalgia	80	42	25		29	20	23
Irritable bowel syndrome	55	50	27	43		26	27
Chronic fatigue syndrome	45	49	26	36	32		13
Chronic pelvic pain	34	51	25	53	44	17	

TTH, tension-type headache; NCCP, non-cardiac chest pain; FM, fibromyalgia; IBS, irritable bowel syndrome; CFS, chronic fatigue syndrome; CPP, chronic pelvic pain.

is substantial overlap – and that patients with symptoms of one syndrome commonly have additional symptoms of another. This was mentioned in Chapter 1 and is elaborated in Table 2.2, which shows the overlap of a range of functional syndromes among patients referred to one of six specialist clinics.

Epidemiological associations of MUS

MUS are more common in women than in men and there is a socioeconomic gradient, with MUS more common in patients with poorer socioeconomic status. MUS tends to run in families, although it is not clear how much this is due to genes, shared adversity or learned behaviours. Adversity, particularly in childhood, is a predisposing factor, particularly for the most severely affected patients in whom a history of abuse is relatively common. Among all the risk factors, it seems that none is either sufficient or necessary for the development of MUS and, particularly in the case of prior abuse, it seems better to be prepared if a patient wishes to discuss this, rather than to go looking.

Impact of MUS

Quality of life

Patients with MUS are sometimes portrayed as the 'worried well', but this is generally not the case. Studies of health-related quality of life in patients with multiple MUS (the 2% of consulters) consistently show that their quality of life is impaired – often to the same level as patients with comparable rates of attendance and referral for 'explained' symptoms. Pain, fatigue, limitation of activities and difficulty performing tasks are all common physical components of impaired quality of life. Anxiety and depression are both more common in patients with MUS (as they are in people with explained illness) but this is not invariably the case. These too impair patients quality of life.

Healthcare usage and costs

Patients with MUS symptoms use a substantial proportion of healthcare resources. One recent estimate put the cost of MUS to the UK NHS at around £3.1 billion per year. Compared with patients with explained illness, patients with MUS have more investigations (perhaps because one negative investigation is followed by another). However, when referred, they are less likely to be followed up in specialist care than patients with explained symptoms and more likely just to be discharged back to the GP.

The increased costs among MUS patients are not limited to those most severely affected; indeed because there are more of them, moderately affected patients with MUS (that 2% of the practice population again) account for a similar volume of healthcare usage to the small number of more severe cases. Mental health costs do not seem to be increased in patients with MUS.

Conclusion

MUS are very common in primary and secondary care. They have a substantial impact on health services and on the patients themselves.

Further reading

Burton C, McGorm K, Richardson G, Weller D, Sharpe M. Health care costs incurred by patients repeatedly referred to secondary care with medically unexplained symptoms: a case control study. *J Psychosom Res* 2012;**72**:242–7.

McGorm K, Burton C, Weller D, Murray G, Sharpe M. Patients repeatedly referred to secondary care with symptoms unexplained by organic disease: prevalence, characteristics and referral pattern. *Fam Pract* 2010;**27**:479–86.

Nimnuan C, Hotopf M, Wessely S. Medically unexplained symptoms: an epidemiological study in seven specialities. *J Psychosom Res* 2001;**51**:361–7.

Verhaak PF, Meijer SA, Visser AP, Wolters G. Persistent presentation of medically unexplained symptoms in general practice. *Fam Pract* 2006;**23**:414–20.

CHAPTER 3

Considering Organic Disease

David Weller[1] and Chris Burton[2]

[1]Centre for Population Health Sciences, University of Edinburgh, Edinburgh, UK
[2]University of Aberdeen, Aberdeen, UK

OVERVIEW

- Symptoms that appear to be functional will sometimes turn out to indicate serious illness
- Premature closure of diagnostic reasoning and failure to consider the possibility of serious disease are the commonest serious diagnostic errors
- Errors of judgement and system failures are far more common than errors due to lack of knowledge

---

Introduction

Every patient who presents with a medically unexplained symptom (MUS) will eventually die, and many of them will consult a doctor with symptoms of their final illness. This sobering thought is the reason for this chapter, which aims to highlight particular problems and pitfalls when managing functional symptoms. A long history of MUS, particularly when combined with frequent attendance, can sometimes distract clinicians from one of their core tasks – diagnosing serious illness.

The chapter aims to answer three questions: how commonly does the diagnoses of MUS need to be revised; what are the factors associated with practitioner delay in diagnosing cancer; and what are the commonest diagnostic errors made by doctors.

This chapter does not list specific sets of red flags–they are described in individual chapters – but several themes are consistent across symptoms and body systems. Bleeding is never a symptom of MUS; similarly unintentional weight loss and night sweats need investigation – sometimes extensive investigation – to look for disease.

Symptom-specific recommendations for investigations are also included in the relevant chapters. However, as a rule of thumb, most non-trivial new symptoms in a patient who has not had recent investigations warrant basic blood tests: full blood count, renal, liver, thyroid and bone chemistry and inflammatory marker – with more added as clinically indicated. There is little evidence that deferring investigations is better or worse than carrying them out

on the first occasion the patient presents with potentially significant symptoms.

How commonly does MUS turn out to be organic disease?

Surprisingly few studies have reported this. One small UK study found that in primary care, 10% of symptoms that have been present for several months and were thought to be MUS turned out to be due to organic disease. In secondary care the proportion is smaller, especially when the specialist concludes that there is a functional disorder rather than the diagnosis remaining ambiguous. A diagnosis of functional symptoms from a neurologist turns out to be wrong in only 2–3% of cases and similar proportions are probably seen by specialists in other disciplines.

New symptoms that are accompanied by anxiety are especially challenging, particularly when the patient has a past history of anxiety or panic disorder. Anxiety is one of a range of factors that may raise the practitioner's threshold of suspicion regarding new symptoms and which may inhibit timely recognition, diagnosis and referral. This kind of parallel presentation does not mean that recognition and treatment of the psychological disorder is unimportant, rather it acts as a reminder that the two can coexist.

What are the factors associated with practitioner delay in diagnosing serious illness?

Practitioner delay has been studied most thoroughly in relation to cancer diagnosis and the evidence for this has recently been exhaustively reviewed. The effect of patients' sociodemographic characteristics has a variable effect on practitioner delay.

Patient characteristics

Patient age is a factor in delayed cancer diagnosis, particularly for gastrointestinal cancers. Younger patients are at greater risk of diagnostic delay. Although this is perhaps understandable – the probability that a new disorder is functional is higher in younger patients – it is a salutary reminder of the need to consider the possibility of organic disease. Practitioners need to be alert to the possibility of patients presenting outside 'typical' age

ABC of Medically Unexplained Symptoms, First Edition.
Edited by Christopher Burton.

ranges – the young patient presenting with a familial colorectal cancer is a classic example. Diagnostic delay of urological, gynaecological and lung cancer is associated with lower educational attainment in patients, perhaps because of lower health literacy or because of greater reluctance to challenge the doctor's (incorrect) opinion. Recent evidence based on audit of cases of cancer referrals suggests that patients who are housebound may experience longer delays; multiple comorbidity may also lead to longer diagnostic intervals. In general the more complex the 'background' level of symptoms, the more likely it is that a diagnosis might be delayed.

Patient healthcare behaviour

Frequent healthcare seeking and seeing multiple providers – as is the case for some patients with MUS – are associated with greater delay in diagnosis of gynaecological and colorectal cancers. It is important to remember that patients with MUS have the same risk of serious illness as those without MUS. Practitioners need to be vigilant and monitor the pattern of presentation, looking particularly for subtle changes that might signal an emerging organic illness.

Practitioner response

Diagnostic delay due to practitioner response is associated with errors of judgement, including incorrect diagnosis, or symptomatic treatment without a clear diagnosis. It is also associated with errors of procedure such as inadequate examination, failure to organise tests and failure to ensure adequate follow-up of patients or tests. Importantly, it appears that diagnostic delay is reduced – at least in gastrointestinal cancer – by following referral guidelines.

Health system factors

Factors such as short consultation times and lack of access to diagnostic investigations can also lead to prolonged diagnostic intervals. In primary care we typically place great store in continuity of care – that is, seeing the same doctor on a regular basis. Although the benefits of continuity of care have been well described, there is at least anecdotal evidence that sometimes a 'fresh pair of eyes' can shed a different light on a difficult diagnosis. There is probably a case for encouraging long standing MUS patients with complex symptoms to see more than one practitioner over prolonged periods. The gatekeeper role of primary care is also widely supported yet we should keep an open mind about whether it might itself lead to delays in diagnosis; indeed there is some evidence that countries with strong gatekeeper systems have longer intervals to a diagnosis of cancer.

What are the commonest diagnostic errors?

Apart from the work on cancer, there has been relatively little research on diagnostic errors specific to primary care. However, more general work on errors has been carried out, especially in the USA. Although the relative incidence of errors may not be transferrable to UK primary care it is nonetheless worthwhile examining the common errors.

The commonest error in several series is failure to consider the diagnosis. There are several possible mechanisms for this and the cognitive processing errors that underpin these are described below.

Other common causes of diagnostic error include failure to order tests (either by not ordering or through logistical error) and difficulties with interpretation of results (including false negative results). Less common, although still important, are errors in history taking (failure to elicit the critical piece of information) and examination (omitting the critical element). Errors of judgement between two diagnoses occur but are not among the most common errors reported by doctors. Strikingly, in this and other studies of medical error, lack of knowledge is rarely the main problem.

Misdiagnosis is the most common factor in medical litigation cases in primary care. It is rare for such cases to identify significant knowledge deficits among practitioners; more typically misdiagnosis is found to be associated with poor communication, procedural errors, and failure to consider more serious diagnoses in the background of multiple, vague, or atypical symptom presentations.

Cognitive processing errors

Practitioners typically use a hypothetico-deductive model in reaching diagnoses. This model relies on selective enquiry as various avenues of diagnosis are explored until the practitioner is satisfied he/she has reached a conclusion that matches the presentation. Of course, this relies on quite complex cognitive processes and many errors appear to be underpinned by problems in the way clinicians process information. These are human characteristics that have been classified as cognitive processing errors. Awareness of these errors may help clinicians recognise when they are in danger of making them.

Premature closure

This underpins the common diagnostic error of failing to consider the diagnosis. It relates to the point at which the clinician switches from searching for possible diagnoses to deciding that there is sufficient evidence to proceed with the best candidate and stop searching for more information. Interestingly age and experience have little effect on premature closure and it appears to be a characteristic of some doctors' problem-solving style.

Availability bias

People tend to overestimate the frequency of easily remembered events and underestimate the frequency of ordinary or uninteresting events. Unusual clinical cases are more memorable than routine ones and so may lead doctors to overlook the ordinary and unremarkable diagnoses. Availability bias is one of the reasons doctors are repeatedly taught that 'canaries' are usually just 'sparrows'.

Representativeness bias

Clinicians naturally try to fit cases to the most typical condition. Although this seems like an efficient pattern-matching approach, it often operates independently of rules of probability. This has two implications: first if the best-fitting diagnosis is a rare condition and a nearly fitting diagnosis is common, then the nearly fitting common diagnosis is more likely, but representativeness bias will argue the other way. Second, when one feature (for instance a red flag symptom) is strongly indicative of a serious condition but nothing else quite fits, the doctor may ignore it when the remaining symptoms fit better with an alternative diagnosis.

Anchoring and conservatism

As clinicians build up the evidence in order to solve a diagnostic problem, the natural tendency is to stick to the first hypothesis and test information against this. This 'anchoring' on the first hypothesis leads to conservatism as new information is gathered. In turn, new information that fits the anchor is more likely to be retained whereas that which points to another diagnosis will be ignored or discarded.

Scenario 1

'Richard' is a 55-year-old man with a history of depression and of panic attacks but not of bowel symptoms. He has been seeing the GP over recent months with low mood and anxiety following the breakup of his marriage. He has sometimes reported vague symptoms including headaches, palpitations and sweatiness although these have typically resolved spontaneously. During one appointment he mentions that he is getting worried by bloating and rumbling in his abdomen and the GP considers that his symptoms are all in keeping with this. At the end of the consultation, Richard mentions a little bit of rectal bleeding which was 'probably just haemorrhoids' and the GP, who is writing up the consultation, agrees.

Richard doesn't mention his gastrointestinal symptoms at the next two consultations even though they have continued. The consultations have focused on his anxiety and depression and his requests for sickness leave. Eight months later he presents to the emergency department with obstruction due to a sigmoid carcinoma.

Principles for safe practice with suspected MUS

- Use the history to check for red-flag symptoms and record that you have asked about them.
- Carry out (and document) a careful but focused examination.
- Be familiar with referral guidelines, and unless you can clearly justify it, adhere to them.

- Investigate new symptoms if non-trivial or persistent unless the patient is a particularly frequent presenter.
- Ensure you have systems in place for appropriate follow-up of patients and tests (including negative tests).
- Have a policy of deliberately re-thinking the diagnosis if the clinical picture is not progressing as you would expect.
- Consider adopting a 'safety netting' approach in which you systematically re-visit uncertain diagnoses and provide clear guidance to your patients that they should return for review if symptoms persist.
- Be aware that patients may misinterpret the advice you provide about their symptoms. They may mistake your guarded assurance with 'safety netting' for complete reassurance and fail to take further action if their symptoms persist or worsen. Repetition and documentation of advice can be helpful in this case.

Summary

Patient with presumed MUS have a low (but not negligible) probability of serious disease. Guidelines exist for common situations (such as dyspepsia and suspected IBS) that take a reasonable balance between under- and overinvestigation. In other situations, awareness of the common sources of diagnostic error and cognitive processing errors that underpin them can lead to safer practice.

Further reading

Macleod U, Mitchell ED, Burgess C, Macdonald S, Ramirez AJ. Risk factors for delayed presentation and referral of symptomatic cancer: evidence for common cancers. *Br J Cancer* 2009;**101**(Suppl 2):S92–S101.

Elstein AS, Schwarz A. Clinical problem solving and diagnostic decision making: selective review of the cognitive literature. *BMJ* 2002; **324**:729–32.

Vedsted P, Olesen F. Are the serious problems in cancer survival partly rooted in gatekeeper principles? An ecologic study. *Br J Gen Pract* 2011;**61**(589):e508–12.

Hamilton W. Cancer diagnosis in primary care. *Br J Gen Pract* 2010;**60**(571):121–8.

Hamilton W. The CAPER studies: five case–control studies aimed at identifying and quantifying the risk of cancer in symptomatic primary care patients. *Br J Cancer* 2009;**101**(2):S80–6.

Almond S, Mant D, Thompson M. Diagnostic safety-netting. *Br J Gen Pract* 2009;**59**(568):872–4; discussion 874.

Rubin G. National audit of cancer diagnosis in primary care. http://www.dur.ac.uk/resources/school.health/erdu /NationalAuditofCancerDiagnosisinPrimaryCare.pdf.

CHAPTER 4

Considering Depression and Anxiety

Alan Carson[1] and Jon Stone[2]

[1]Robert Fergusson Unit, University of Edinburgh, Edinburgh, UK
[2]Department of Clinical Neurosciences, Western General Hospital, Edinburgh, UK

OVERVIEW

- Depression and anxiety are common in patients with medically unexplained symptoms (MUS); most patients have elements of both
- MUS are not the same as depression and anxiety, although MUS predispose to emotional disorder and emotional disorders predispose to MUS
- Many patients with MUS will play down their emotional symptoms for fear of being mislabelled
- Questionnaires such as the Patient Health Questionnaire (PHQ9) and Generalized Anxiety Disorder scale (GAD7) or Hospital Anxiety and Depression Scale (HADS) can help patients see that their emotions are typical of depression or anxiety

Introduction

In this chapter we outline a clinical approach to the detection and assessment of depressive and anxiety disorders. Treatment is covered separately in Chapters 15–17.

Epidemiology

Major depressive disorder, diagnosed using standard criteria (see Box 4.1) is common in the general population and in patients with MUS. Typical population-based studies suggest a prevalence of around 2% with a lifetime incidence of 6–9% for women and 3–5% for men. It occurs across all ages with a peak incidence at around 40 years old.

Box 4.1 Major depressive episode (proposed criteria DSM 5)

A. Five (or more) of the following criteria have been present during the same 2-week period and represent a change from previous functioning; at least one of the symptoms is either (1) depressed mood or (2) loss of interest or pleasure

1 Depressed mood most of the day, nearly every day, as indicated by either subjective report (e.g., feels sad or empty) or observation made by others (e.g., appears tearful). Note: In children and adolescents, can be irritable mood

2 Markedly diminished interest or pleasure in all, or almost all, activities most of the day, nearly every day (as indicated by either subjective account or observation made by others)

3 Significant weight loss when not dieting or weight gain (e.g., a change of more than 5% of body weight in a month), or decrease or increase in appetite nearly every day. Note: In children, consider failure to make expected weight gain

4 Insomnia or hypersomnia nearly every day

5 Psychomotor agitation or retardation nearly every day (observable by others, not merely subjective feelings of restlessness or being slowed down)

6 Fatigue or loss of energy nearly every day

7 Feelings of worthlessness or excessive or inappropriate guilt (which may be delusional) nearly every day (not merely self-reproach or guilt about being sick)

8 Diminished ability to think or concentrate, or indecisiveness, nearly every day (either by subjective account or as observed by others)

9 Recurrent thoughts of death (not just fear of dying), recurrent suicidal ideation without a specific plan, or a suicide attempt or a specific plan for committing suicide

Generalised anxiety disorder (Box 4.2) has a prevalence of 3-4% in woman and 2–3% in men. The prevalence of panic disorder (1%) (Box 4.3) and phobic disorders (1–2%) is slightly lower.

Box 4.2 Generalized Anxiety Disorder (proposed criteria DSM 5)

A. Excessive anxiety and worry (apprehensive expectation) about two (or more) domains of activities or events (for example, domains like family, health, finances, and school/work difficulties)

B. The excessive anxiety and worry occur on more days than not for 3 months or more

ABC of Medically Unexplained Symptoms, First Edition.
Edited by Christopher Burton.

C. The anxiety and worry are associated with one or more of the following symptoms:

1 Restlessness or feeling keyed up or on edge
2 Being easily fatigued
3 Difficulty concentrating or mind going blank
4 Irritability
5 Muscle tension
6 Sleep disturbance (difficulty falling or staying asleep, or restless unsatisfying sleep)

D. The anxiety and worry are associated with one (or more) of the following behaviors:

1 Marked avoidance of situations in which a negative outcome could occur
2 Marked time and effort preparing for situations in which a negative outcome could occur
3 Marked procrastination in behavior or decision-making due to worries
4 Repeatedly seeking reassurance due to worries

Box 4.3 **Panic Disorder (proposed criteria DSM 5)**

A. Recurrent unexpected panic attacks defined as: a discrete period of intense fear or discomfort, in which four (or more) of the following symptoms developed abruptly and reached a peak within 10 minutes: 1) palpitations, pounding heart, or accelerated heart rate; 2) sweating; 3) trembling or shaking; 4) sensations of shortness of breath or smothering; 5) feeling of choking; 6) chest pain or discomfort; 7) nausea or abdominal distress; 8) feeling dizzy, unsteady, lightheaded, or faint; 9) derealization (feelings of unreality) or depersonalization (being detached from oneself); 10) fear of losing control or going crazy; 11) fear of dying; 12) paresthesias (numbness or tingling sensations); 13) chills or hot flushes

B. At least one of the attacks has been followed by 1 month (or more) of one or both of the following:

1 Persistent concern or worry about additional panic attacks or their consequences (e.g., losing control, having a heart attack, going crazy).
2 Significant maladaptive change in behavior related to the attacks (e.g., behaviors designed to avoid having panic attacks, such as avoidance of exercise or unfamiliar situations).

However, these psychiatric definitions of depressive and anxiety disorders were developed in secondary care where only a small proportion of those with symptoms of any of the emotional disorders are seen. At a population level the presence of symptoms of emotional disorder is continuously distributed (Figure 4.1) and the classical psychiatric diagnostic categories have limited value. In primary care most patients present with a mixed picture of anxiety and depression and meet the criteria for more than one diagnosis. Taken as a group depressive and anxiety disorders have a prevalence of around 10% in women and 5% in men.

Depression and anxiety are more common in patients with MUS. Approximately three-quarters of patients with significant MUS will

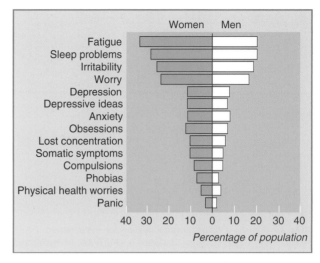

Figure 4.1 Symptoms of depressive and anxiety disorders are continuously distributed in the population. Reprinted from Mayou R, Sharpe M, Carson A. (2003) A*BC of Psychological Medicine*. BMJ books, with permission from John Wiley & Sons Ltd.

report symptoms of depression and/or anxiety; this is about twice the rate in patients with equivalent physical disability from organic disease. As the severity of MUS increase so does the likelihood and the severity of emotional disorder.

This has led to a view of the emotional disorder as the cause of the physical symptoms – so called somatisation of distress. In turn this has led to the idea that treatment should be by reattribution of the symptoms back to a psychological cause. However, this view may be wrong: the correlation of any two given symptoms (e.g. pain and fatigue) tends to show a similar relationship. In practice, it may be incorrect, as well as unhelpful to assume causal directions for these interrelationships. Longitudinal studies suggest that symptoms and emotional disorders are each a risk factor for the other.

Diagnosis

Depression

You should base the diagnosis of emotional disorders on a combination of history and examination of mental state. The typical patient with depression, feels down, tearful and lethargic. This is accompanied by a cognitive triad of distorted mind-sets with thoughts of hopelessness and futility about the future, a sense of worthlessness about the present and a sense of guilt about the past. The symptom of anhedonia, the inability to experience pleasure, is central. There is usually a range of somatic symptoms including disturbed sleep with early morning wakening and lack of refreshment, loss of appetite, poor concentration, loss of libido and a sense of general malaise.

In patients who present with such overt mood symptoms the diagnostic challenge is to separate out those in whom this represents new symptoms from those who have dysthymic personalities by asking

'when did this first start?', 'have you always been like this since you were a teenager?', 'is this a change from your normal self?'.

In many patients with MUS detection is less straightforward. Patients may emphasise the somatic element of the presentation and

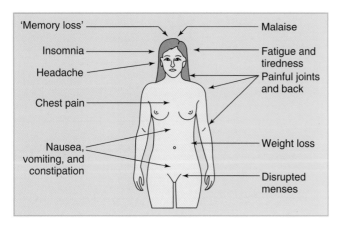

Figure 4.2 Somatic complaints raising the suspicion of depression. Reprinted from Mayou R, Sharpe M, Carson A. (2003) A*BC of Psychological Medicine*. BMJ books, with permission from John Wiley & Sons Ltd.

view mood symptoms as a rational response to intolerable physical symptoms rather than an illness in its own right. The presence of low mood may be denied in response to direct questions, partly because the patient is aware that the doctor is 'angling' for a psychiatric diagnosis. Exploring mood in this situation requires considerable tact. When suspicion is raised due to the presence of typical somatic symptoms (Figure 4.2) sympathetic, leading questions can be more fruitful.

It must be difficult living with all that pain . . . Have you cut down on your range of activities? . . . .

Do you find you stopped enjoying things that you can still manage to do physically? . . .

What about watching your favourite programme on TV?, do you still enjoy it?

When friends or relatives come to visit do you look forward to their company as a break from the monotony? . . . or do you just want to hide away and wish they would go?

Generalised and phobic anxiety

The core of an anxiety disorder is disproportionate, persistent and unwelcome worry. Anxiety disorders present with a range of somatic symptoms such as muscle tension/pain, fatigue, tingling, nausea and poor concentration (Figure 4.3), and symptoms associated with excessive, shallow or disordered breathing. Abdominal bloating and borborygmi, from aerophagy, are common. Peripheral paraethesiae affecting fingertips, toes and perioral regions, are common but tetany is rare. Patients will often report sensory symptoms as unilateral, but on questioning will usually disclose very mild symptoms on the opposite side. Patients often complain of fluid sensations under their scalp or tightly localised, transient headache that they 'can put a finger on'. Commonly, anxiety tends to exacerbate existing primary headache disorders such as migraine.

Where anxiety disorders are suspected the key distinction is to separate generalised anxiety, which presents with ruminative worry about a wide range of topics with no consistency or theme, from

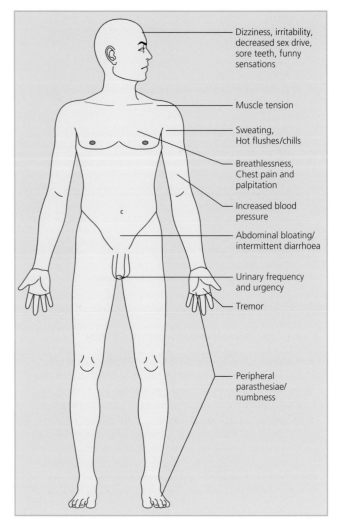

Figure 4.3 Somatic complaints raising the suspicion of anxiety.

phobic anxiety, in which anxiety presents in response to a given stimulus. Phobic anxiety, and its associated symptoms, will begin in anticipation of the stimulus (which may be going out, or the onset of a symptom), build to a peak after the start of the trigger and then subside: either quickly if the patient 'escapes', or more slowly if the patient 'sits it out' and learns that they can master the anxiety. As these behaviours are learned, each time the patient 'escapes to safety' the behaviour is reinforced, and the anxiety escalates for the next time. Conversely learning to 'sit it out' reduces anxiety over time.

In patients with MUS a phobic component of anxiety may be obscured by misattribution to physical disease. This can follow an agoraphobic pattern in which 'attacks' attributed to effort occur on leaving the house 'my heart beats like crazy, my legs turn to jelly, I feel I am going to collapse, I just have to sit down, I can only manage to walk 200 yards before it happens'. Alternatively the fear may be of a symptom: 'bringing on pain' and 'falling' are both common. This leads to cycles of decreased activity that can in turn lead to physiological complications through disuse (for more information on explaining cycles of perpetuating factors see Chapters 15 and 16).

As with depression, be careful asking questions about anxiety in patients with MUS – there is a risk they will see you as criticising them personally or labelling them a 'hypochondriac'. Useful questions include:

Do you often find yourself feeling worried about your symptoms?

Do you often feel on edge or tense about things?

Do you ever feel like you can't keep a lid on that worry?

Do you ever get lots of physical symptoms all at once?

Is it frightening when that happens?

Family history, childhood and recent stress

Depression and anxiety are multifactorial in aetiology. Genes may play a part, so consider a family history from that perspective. Childhood adverse experiences predispose to depressive and anxiety disorders conditions in adult life. Enquiry here needs to be tactful and if it is the first time you have discussed emotional distress with the patient it may be best left for a subsequent occasion. Treatment of MUS does not need patients to disclose every abusive experience – indeed in many circumstances that may be actively unhelpful. What one wishes to gain is some general overview of childhood. If the patient discloses, or hints strongly at, significant physical or sexually abusive experiences it is often more helpful to let them set the pace of any disclosure rather than to push the issue: 'is that something you would be able to tell me a bit more about or is it something you would prefer to pass over for now?'. More commonly however the aversive experiences are milder – questions such as:

Did you feel secure and cared for as a child? Did you feel a burden to your parents?

Did you get bullied at school.

What was the atmosphere like at home? . . . did you parents argue a lot? . . . did they ever hit each other?

Did either of your parents drink too much?

Recent life events and stressors are also important and in general, patients are more forthcoming in this area. Indeed, recordings of GP consultations suggest that patients volunteer such explanations for their physical symptoms and doctors close down such enquires too early in a rush to exclude biomedical causes of disease.

Patient:	*The pain is just kind of all over.*
GP:	*And when does it come on?*
Patient:	*It started shortly after my divorce.*
GP:	*And is it there through the night, are you OK generally, weight steady, no night sweats?*

Some patients, however, will flatly deny any problems in their life even though you sense that they may be distressed by their personal circumstances. This can be difficult to deal with; challenging them usually just makes the patient defensive. Patience is usually the key, so keep a mental note that it is a subject to return to. Occasionally the unexpected 'You're getting all these severe stomach pains, you've been off work for 6 weeks and you are not worried – I would be!!' pays dividends.

Suicide and self-harm

When the diagnosis of a significant emotional disorder is made, a brief enquiry about suicidal thought or behaviour is mandatory. You may feel embarrassed about asking about suicide in this situation. In reality, for someone considering ending their life one or two gentle questions is likely to be the least of their problems. In fact most suicidal patients welcome polite enquiry and perhaps counter-intuitively are generally open and honest in their replies; few patients 'cry wolf'. Vague existential worries about 'is it all worthwhile?' are quite common in the population but specific ideas of suicide should always be taken seriously and actual plans should be regarded as a potential emergency. The more lethal and specific the method the more concern should be raised.

Self-harming behaviour is often different from suicidal behaviour. Overdosing is often used as a form of problem solving and self-cutting as a maladaptive means of relieving psychological tension. However, the two do overlap and patients who self-harm have a 100-fold increased rate of completed suicide. They can pose major management problem and specialist advice and help is often required.

Patients' beliefs

In the patient with MUS who also has anxiety or depression, it is vital to understand their perspective. The patient may offer a psychological explanation ('I was really just putting it down to my working an 80-hour week') a physical one ('I'm sure this must be something serious like multiple sclerosis or cancer'), or something in-between. If you know your patient's starting point, you can orient the explanation of the emotional disorder accordingly. Patients with MUS vary in whether they regard low mood as a depressive illness or as an understandable reaction to their illness. In terms of anxiety, most see themselves as cautious or even a bit of a worrier but contrast this with others who may be 'neurotic' or 'a hypochondriac'.

Questionnaires

As a GP, you will be familiar with at least one of the short depression questionnaires such as the Patent Health Questionnaire 9 items (PHQ 9), Hospital Anxiety and Depression Scale (HADS) or the Beck Depression Inventory (BDI). The HADS is the only one that includes anxiety but the other two come with matching anxiety measures: the Generalized Anxiety Disorder 7 item (GAD7) and the Beck Anxiety Inventory. There is little evidence to suggest that any one is superior, and they all tend to overdiagnose emotional disorder if used literally. They are designed to screen for or confirm clinical diagnoses, but are not sufficient to make a diagnosis by themselves. They can, however, be useful for drawing attention to the patient's problems during clinical assessment.

Investigations

Emotional symptoms can be the presenting symptoms of a disease process. Any new onset emotional disorder should be investigated although in most circumstances this can be limited to a small number of routine blood test – full blood count, ferritin, urea and electrolytes, liver function tests including gamma-glutamyl transferase (gamma GT), an inflammatory marker, thyroid function tests, calcium and blood glucose. Further investigations may be appropriate depending on the clinical picture.

Explaining the diagnosis

Once a diagnosis has been made it is important to tell the patient about it. Many doctors feel awkward about this. However, mumbling euphemisms while avoiding eye contact is unlikely to help anyone and certainly will not destigmatise anything.

Somewhat bizarrely many clinicians approach the explanation of the diagnosis by asking the patient what they think may be wrong. This is an important question but, should already have been asked during history taking and not left to the end of the consultation. The patient has come to see you because of your expert knowledge. A simple and effective approach is to treat emotional disorders as any other disease and explain clearly, in language appropriate to the patient, what the diagnosis is and why you think that, then to discuss together what can be done. Patients may find their results on questionnaires such as the PHQ9 and GAD7 a valuable confirmation of the doctor's impression: indicating that they "tick all the boxes".

Further reading

American Psychiatric Association. *Diagnostic and Statistical Manual of Mental Disorders (DSM-5)*. Available at: http://www.dsm5.org (retrieved 26 July 2012).

Kroenke K, Spitzer RL, Williams JB, *et al*. Physical symptoms in primary care. Predictors of psychiatric disorders and functional impairment. *Arch Fam Med* 1994;**3**:774–9.

Lowe B, Spitzer RL, Williams JB, Mussell M, Schellberg D, Kroenke K. Depression, anxiety and somatization in primary care: syndrome overlap and functional impairment. *Gen Hosp Psychiatry* 2008;**30**:191–9.

Mayou R, Sharpe M, Carson A. *ABC of Psychological Medicine*. BMJ Books, London, 2003.

PHQ Questionnaires (contains the PHQ9, GAD7 and PHQ15 questionnaires). Available at: http://www.phqscreeners.com/ (retrieved 26 July 2012).

CHAPTER 5

Medically Unexplained Symptoms and the General Practitioner

Christopher Dowrick

Department of Mental and Behavioural Health Sciences, University of Liverpool, Liverpool, UK

OVERVIEW

- Medically unexplained symptoms (MUS) are a source of diagnostic confusion for GPs
- MUS can be frustrating for GPs and for patients
- The main expectation of patients with MUS is for support and an explanation from their GP, rather than cure
- Our responses to patients presenting with MUS sometimes make the situation worse
- We need to live with uncertainty, while acknowledging suffering, and offering tangible explanations and hope

---

MUS and diagnostic confusion

MUS are a source of great diagnostic confusion for GPs. This is not simply because, by definition, they are symptoms for which no pathophysiological cause is readily identifiable. It is also because of uncertain case definition and variable clinical context.

Uncertain case definition

There is disagreement between clinical authorities as to how MUS should best be understood (Box 5.1). Physicians see them as functional syndromes, related to their sphere of expertise: IBS for gastroenterologists, fibromyalgia for rheumatologists, non-cardiac chest pain for cardiologists, and so on. Many psychiatrists see them as somatisation disorders, manifestations of underlying mental disorders such as anxiety or depression, although they disagree among themselves about the precise ways in which somatisation disorders should be classified. Psychologists may focus on symptom amplification, referring to a patient's tendency to attribute amplified or exaggerated symptoms such as pain or distress to a presenting problem such as osteoarthritis of the knee. Health service researchers focus on problems of frequent attendance in primary care, or excessive referrals to secondary care and the wasteful costs to the healthcare system which ensue. Other researchers, including me, focus on problems in communication between patients and health professionals.

ABC of Medically Unexplained Symptoms, First Edition.
Edited by Christopher Burton.
© 2013 John Wiley & Sons, Ltd. Published 2013 by John Wiley & Sons, Ltd.

Box 5.1 **Uncertain case definition**

- Functional syndromes
- Somatoform disorders
- Symptom amplification
- Healthcare misuse
- Communication problems

Variable clinical context

The clinical context within which patients present with MUS can vary considerably (see Box 5.2). In primary care patients commonly present with several symptoms, each of which may have a different degree of medical explicability. MUS may occur in the context of confirmed disease, whether physical or psychiatric. Medical explicability may also vary over time. In about 10% of symptom presentations initially considered as unexplained, a pathophysiological diagnosis becomes apparent within the following 12 months. Conversely, symptoms that appear to be clearly attributable to a recognised disease process can persist even when tests indicate that the assumed disease process is not present.

Box 5.2 **Variations in clinical context of MUS**

- Multiple symptom presentation
- With differing degrees of explicability
- Explained and unexplained symptoms may co-exist
- Explicability may vary over time
- Unexplained symptoms may become explained
- Current explanations may be disproved

Let us consider how this confusion affects our understanding of the problems presented by 'Frank', a 38-year-old plumber.

If Frank sees a gastroenterologist he is likely to receive a diagnosis of IBS. If he is interviewed by a psychiatrist, he might fit criteria for DSM-IV somatoform disorder. His symptoms are not fully explained by a general medical condition, the direct effect of drugs or another mental disorder; they cause him clinically significant distress, and lead to impairment of social, occupational and other

Scenario 1

'Frank' consults you about his stomach pain. He says he finds it hard to pin down exactly where it is. It starts with his tummy button but spreads all over one side. It has been off and on for the past 2 years, and this is the eleventh time he's consulted your or one of your colleagues about it. It lasts around a day at a time, sometimes longer. He finds it hard to get to sleep because he has to try to lie in a way that eases the pain. When it flares up he feels very low, thinking 'oh no, this is starting again'. When it's not happening he feels anxious that that it might start again. A previous doctor suggested he had bruised his ribs. Another doctor had suggested gall-stones. He has had blood tests and scans of his gall-bladder and liver, but these were all normal.

He has found himself noticing other problems lately, although he is not sure whether you will have time to hear about them as well as his stomach pain. He had a migraine the other day. He used to get them a lot but has been free of them for a few years. He has also had bad acne for about 3 months. Whatever he does, the spots won't go away. He has a mole on his arm which might have grown a little over the last few months. At night he has throbbing in his leg sometimes. He is worried what it all might be.

areas of functioning. He does not fulfil criteria for full somatisation disorder: for this he would need to complain of at least 12 different symptoms over many years. However, he does meet criteria for abridged somatisation disorder, since he presents with at least four somatic symptoms. He may meet diagnostic criteria for an anxiety disorder, and possibly for major depression. A psychologist would focus on Frank's symptom behaviours, particularly his fear that his pain is going to get worse.

As a GP, you are aware that he is a frequent attender, and that the costs of investigating his abdominal pain have borne no diagnostic reward.

Then you have the further complexity of the clinical context within which Frank is presenting his abdominal symptoms. His acne is a medically explicable condition, and his migraine probably is too. The mole on his arm may well be benign, but you cannot be sure at this stage. And what about the throbbing in his leg?

The frustration of MUS

GPs often find patients with MUS difficult and frustrating to deal with. We prefer to work with patients who have readily diagnosable problems, whether physical or psychological, for whom there are clear, evidence-based management plans.

Here are some comments that GPs have made about patients presenting with MUS.

Well, you get the chronic ones, coming for years ... the persistent 'nothing makes it better'. The persistent offender, I get really fed up with it.

I find it frustrating in a way ... we go into medicine, perhaps, because we feel we want to help, to do something, then maybe feel we haven't got our pay-off, so what do we do? We get mad with the patient, or impatient with the illness.

It is important to realise that patients with MUS can get equally frustrated with us. The following is a typical comment.

Many times I've come away and I've nearly cried thinking I've gone there and waited, come out and got nowhere.

Many patients are not inclined to accept our assertion that their problems are primarily psychological.

She wasn't getting me – just treating all these little bits separately. She had me written down as a neurotic. She thought it was all me and all in my head. [[Shortly after this, the patient changed her doctor.]]

They fear we will ignore their physical symptoms.

I think once that [[stress]] comes up, they tend to think 'that's it then'.

They may not trust us with discussion of emotional aspects of their problems, and therefore may choose not to present them.

Patients' expectations of GPs

There is a common assumption that patients with MUS are convinced their symptoms have a physical cause, and they come to see their GPs demanding physical solutions. In the great majority of cases, this is not true.

Many patients have thought about what might be causing their symptoms. Their illness models are rich in psychosocial components, and they have considered how these may impact on their physical symptoms.

Most patients with MUS are not expecting their GP to cure them. Instead they are hoping for two things: explanation and support. In the consultation, almost all patients provide opportunities for the GP to address their need for explanation of their symptoms or to have emotional or social problems addressed. The following is a common example.

But I just don't know, but all of a sudden they're really, really. Honest to God it's a nightmare sometimes.

How GPs can make the situation worse

GPs often try to contain the situation by normalisation, stressing to the patient that there is no serious disease, that symptoms are likely to be benign or self-limiting, and that there is no need for healthcare intervention. However if we are not careful, our responses can be ineffective, or exacerbate patients' presentations. Box 5.3 gives examples of ineffective normalisation strategies.

These strategies tend to be counterproductive. Patients respond by providing further evidence for the importance of their problems, elaborating their symptoms or introducing external authority for them; or by expressing uncertainty or concern; or introducing new symptoms.

Although patients with MUS present with a variety of problems and cues, GPs are more likely to pay attention to their physical symptoms than to their psychological or social problems. We are also more likely than our patients to propose investigations, somatic treatments or referrals. As a result, we encourage the persistence of MUS in our patients.

Box 5.3 **Ineffective normalisation**

Normalisation without explanation

- Dismissal of disease: 'I don't think there's anything serious going on'
- Rudimentary reassurance: 'It will settle, it's just a matter of time'
- Authority of negative test result: 'Anyway, your scan showed nothing wrong'

Normalisation with ineffective explanation

- Tangible physical mechanism, unrelated to patient's concerns: 'Sometimes stress makes the intestine sensitive'.

Living with uncertainty

GPs are often unsure of the cause of patients' symptoms, or of how best to manage them. It is important for us to recognise, and feel comfortable, with the uncertainty associated with the presentation of MUS in primary care. Successful consultations are likely to contain the key elements shown in Box 5.4.

Box 5.4 **Elements of successful MUS consultations**

- Acknowledge and validate patients' sense of suffering
- Provide tangible mechanisms to explain symptoms, arising from patients' expressed concerns
- Offer opportunity for patients to discuss their psychosocial concerns
- Offer review if symptoms persist or worsen

Returning to Frank, here is an example of how a GP provides a tangible explanation for his abdominal symptoms, and enables him to discuss his psychosocial concerns.

Doctor: *The only thing that fits is, it's the sort of pain you get with shingles because it comes around in that pattern.*
Patient: *Yes, yes.*

Doctor: *And that's sometimes irritation of the nerve endings.*
Patient: *That's what somebody else, me Nan says, 'It could be your nerves'.*
Doctor: *I don't mean your emotional nerves, your actual physical nerves that come round your body – but it could be made worse by stress and things like that.*
Patient: *I mean I'm obviously one of them people that are highly strung anyway, I know that. I'm not, I'm not you know come day go day like a laid back person, I'm quite a, like, you know, everything's got to be done at that day, at that time.*
Doctor: *Have you ever considered/tried any sort of relaxation (therapy) to see if that would help your pain?*

Following this sort of strategy, treating patients with MUS in primary care may become simpler than we think, or fear.

Further reading

Chew-Graham C, May C. Chronic low back pain in general practice: the challenge of the consultation. *Fam Pract* 1999;**16**:46–9.

Chitnis A, Dowrick C, Byng R, Turner P, Shiers D. *Guidance for Health Professionals on Medically Unexplained Symptoms.* Royal College of General Practitioners, London, 2011. Available from: www.rcgp.org.uk/PDF/MUS_guidance_A4_4pp_6.pdf (retrieved 26 July 2012).

Dowrick C, Ring A, Humphris G, Salmon P. Normalisation of unexplained symptoms by general practitioners: a functional typology. *Br J Gen Pract* 2004;**54**:165–70.

Peters S, Rogers A, Salmon P, *et al.* What do patients choose to tell their doctors? Qualitative analysis of potential barriers to reattributing medically unexplained symptoms. *J Gen Intern Med* 2009;**24**:443–9.

Salmon P, Dowrick C, Ring, A, Humphris G. Voiced but unheard agendas: qualitative analysis of the psychosocial cues that patients with unexplained symptoms present to general practitioners. *Br J Gen Pract* 2004;**54**:171–6.

Salmon P, Humphris G, Ring A, Davies, Dowrick C. Primary care consultations about medically unexplained symptoms: the role of patients' presentations and doctors' responses in leading to somatic interventions. *Psychosom Med* 2007;**69**:571–7.

CHAPTER 6

Principles of Assessment and Treatment

Chris Burton

University of Aberdeen, Aberdeen, UK

OVERVIEW

- Listen to the patient
- Consider the possibility of medically unexplained symptoms (MUS) – think about epidemiology and about what is common in particular age groups
- Look for typical clinical features – of both organic disorders and functional (MUS) syndromes
- Target the examination and investigations
- Give a constructive explanation
- Link the explanation to action – either specific or generic
- Set appropriate expectations and safety nets

Introduction

The aim of this chapter is to describe the principles behind identifying, assessing, labelling and managing MUS. These principles will be covered specifically in each of the symptom-specific chapters.

Listening to the patient

As in any field of medicine, eliciting a good patient history is essential in dealing with patients with MUS. Key to this is letting the patient tell their own story as clearly as possible and with the minimum of interruption in the initial stages.

Most patients will have a clear account of their illness in their head as they enter the consulting room. Often it will more or less correspond to the commonsense model of illness. This means the patient will already have considered features such as condition name (or diagnosis), potential causes, timeline, and the likely outcome or treatment. The more you let the patient tell you this for the first one or two minutes of the consultation (using active listening and simple encouragement) the less you will have to get from them later.

As you move to direct questions to clarify what the patient has said, consider getting the patient to describe the experience of the symptom before you pin them down to specifics of time, place

or relationship to other things. Table 6.1 illustrates the difference between asking a patient about the nature and the experience of a symptom.

Notice how the experience of a symptom, elicited with the 'what does it feel like' question can includes emotional or consequential components of the symptom whereas a description of the nature of the symptom is much simpler. Both are of equal value in making a disease diagnosis, but the experiential account gives you greater insight into patient ideas, concerns and expectations without needing to ask additional questions.

Asking when the symptoms first began, or when they were worst, can reveal clues to the diagnosis but there is a need to be careful. A stressful time will increase awareness of anything out of the ordinary including symptoms of serious disease. Furthermore, the patient has control over how they answer this and if a symptom did begin at a stressful time, the patient may wish to disguise this, in case the doctor jumps to conclusions.

You will want to know about patients' ideas, concerns and expectations. Several chapters in this book describe this, but none suggests you bluntly ask 'so what do you think is causing this?' If the patient does not volunteer this – as in the example above – then listen to what the patient is asking you for. If they suggest an explanation, then that is most likely what they want. If they suggest an investigation, then you need to discuss that. Although patients offer cues about what they want, most doctors overestimate patients' wishes for investigation, resulting in unnecessary tests that patients neither want nor need. If you do feel the need to ask

Table 6.1 Difference between asking a patient about the nature and the experience of a symptom.

Describing the nature	Describing the experience
Doctor: *What's the pain like?*	Doctor: *So, what does the pain feel like?*
Patient: *It's a dull ache*	
Doctor: *And when does it come on?*	Patient: *Well it's usually a dull ache, but sometimes it becomes unbearable, you know, as if my back is going to give way*
Patient: *It's really there all the time*	Doctor: *And is there a particular time or place?*
	Patient: *I can usually bear it but I worry when I'm holding my grand-daughter I'll drop her*

ABC of Medically Unexplained Symptoms, First Edition.
Edited by Christopher Burton.
© 2013 John Wiley & Sons, Ltd. Published 2013 by John Wiley & Sons, Ltd.

patients directly about ideas, concerns and expectations then try not to make it confrontational – maybe ask 'so how do you make sense of all these symptoms?' as they are crossing the room to the examination couch. Do not leave it to the end of the consultation, you should have all the information you need before then.

Considering the possibility of MUS

Remember that around one in six patients in a GP clinic will be consulting about symptoms that are not associated with disease. However, it is important to remember also that although most MUS occur in infrequent attenders and do not lead to repeat consultations, around 2% of the population do consult repeatedly with MUS and your records should give you a clue to this. Have they had referrals that resulted in 'no evidence of disease' or one or more symptom syndrome diagnoses such as IBS? Have they had repeated negative investigations, such as thyroid function tests for palpitations and for fatigue? Have they previously been diagnosed with panic disorder (or been seen with panic attacks)?

Look for typical features of organic and functional conditions

Each of the symptom-based chapters in this book aims to point out positive diagnostic features of MUS. MUS do not have to be diagnoses of exclusion (although some exclusion of other things may be necessary); they should be positively sought and assessed. Check also for the important red flags. Unexplained weight loss, night sweats, abnormal bleeding are all signs of disease and not of MUS.

Target your examination and investigations

You do not have time for a detailed examination of everything for every patient so focus. For headaches, check the blood pressure and examine the optic discs. Feel the painful abdomen, listen to the anxious heart. Not to do so diminishes your ability to reassure the patient and help them towards recovery. Remember also that clinical thoroughness and competence is what patients value more than anything else (including prompt appointments and nice doctors).

Whatever body system you are examining there are some important things you can do to add value to your focused examination.

- Be positive about your examination. Avoid the throwaway line of 'let me take a quick look'. An anxious or concerned patient wants a thorough examination. 'Let me take a careful look at this'. 'Good', 'thorough', 'proper' are all useful adjectives for an examination.
- Explain what you are doing. Try to get into the habit of talking patients through some of your examination. This can either be before ('now I want to check there are no swollen glands') or after ('and everything about your abdomen feels normal'). There is no need to describe everything, but some feedback is important and you can target it to areas of specific concern for that patient.

- Report something rather than nothing. 'I've carefully felt your abdomen and there is no sign of any swelling or blockage' is more helpful than 'I can't feel anything'. Again if you listen for patients' concerns before the examination you can address them directly as you examine.
- Point out and explain 'inconsistencies'. Signs such as Hoover's sign (see Chapter 13) or the skin pinch were originally designed to trap patients, however if you demonstrate them, you can use them constructively. If a skin pinch or light touch generates pain (allodynia) then explain how that indicates that the nerves are sending pain signals up to the brain from several healthy areas and not just from one (abnormal) area.

Give constructive explanations

This is probably the thing doctors do least well for patients with MUS. Most explanations given by doctors are either dismissive 'it's nothing serious', or normalising 'it's just a bit of wear and tear', 'it's probably a virus or something'. Some are collusive – 'so, you wonder if you have ME [myalgic encephalomyelitis], well I suppose you might have' and some just bark up the wrong tree 'It's fine, no sign of cancer' – in a patient who wondered whether helicobacter might be causing his dyspepsia.

Constructive explanations have three characteristics: they are plausible and acceptable, they do not imply blame, and they lead to something therapeutic. In addition they should be memorable – a good test is to see if you can summarise the explanation in one or two sentences. If you cannot, then the first time someone asks your patient what you said, you can be certain they will struggle.

Giving constructive explanations is not easy. In addition to the examples in this book, many condition-specific websites have thought long and hard how to describe a condition, so it is worth looking these up. If you wish to make your own explanations then keep them fairly concrete (rather than allegorical) and mechanistic – because that is the way that most people view their body. Spending some time looking up, writing and rehearsing the explanations you give to patients would be a worthwhile piece of reflective practice to include in your appraisal or revalidation portfolio.

Link the explanation to action

In a simple, 'explained' condition, this is easy. 'You have a chest infection, I'm going to prescribe antibiotics for you to take'. In a complicated unexplained condition this is not always so simple. But, as Chapters 15 to 17 clearly demonstrate, whether treatment is cognitive, behavioural or pharmacological, explanation – sometimes with negotiation – is essential. It is illogical to take an antidepressant for physical pain in the pelvis. On the other hand, if the pain is due to nerve circuits that start from the ovaries and surrounding area and are not working properly, then using something to restore these and rebuild the pain barrier makes a lot of sense. Without a constructive explanation, treatment is much less likely to happen. Sometimes the action may be nothing more than a commitment to support the person while they tackle the difficulties you have both identified.

Set appropriate expectations and safety nets

There are two sets of expectations here. Expectations for the symptoms and patients' expectations of you. Both are important.

Expectation of recovery

Most MUS go away. Many go away quite quickly, some take a while, but most resolve. That means that in most cases you can reasonably create an expectation of improvement or recovery. Expectation is one of the key components of the therapeutic effect of consulting a doctor (which underpins the placebo effect) and works in two ways. The first is by converting pessimism to optimism 'The doctor said it will settle' – but that does not last. A second, cognitive, component relates to interpreting change in a positive way. 'She said that to start with there would be the odd good day, and then with time I would start to see more of them. That's happening now so it looks as if I'm on the road to recovery'. Telling patients what you expect of treatment is important for this. But remember that this works the other way too – as discussion of the nocebo effect in Chapter 17 demonstrates.

Expectation of you

Some patients will expect an investigation or referral. If this is their first episode of a new and potentially significant symptom this may be appropriate. If you are not going to investigate then it is important to explain why in a positive way. 'I'm not going to refer you for a scan of your spine because my examination shows there

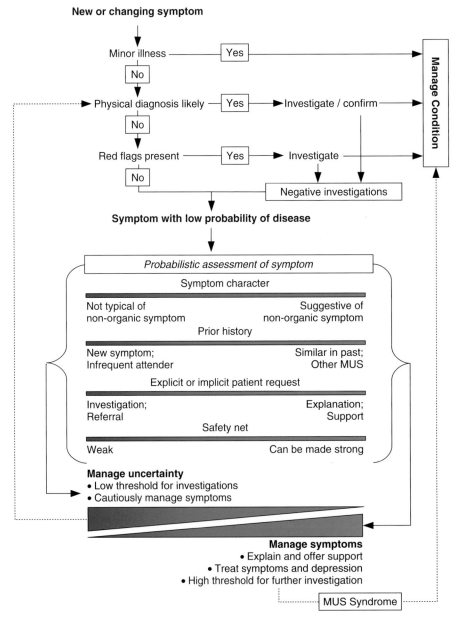

Figure 6.1 Two-stage model evaluating and managing physical symptoms. MUS, medically unexplained symptoms.

are no nerves trapped and a scan can't show which nerves are giving you pain' is better than 'because it will probably be normal'. A few patients will keep requesting investigation or referral, although this is fairly uncommon. In this case you need to have a discussion about what they hope to gain, what they have gained in the past, and why a different way of looking at the problem – based on function rather than structure – is needed. Sometimes pointing out that scans and other tests are 'snapshots' of a system and can never show if something is intact but not working properly can be helpful.

Many patients will hope that you can give them a bit of support as they struggle through a difficult patch. That may be little more than an occasional review, checking that things are stable and some empathic recognition that they are doing OK all things considered. Some patients will be more demanding and for these you may need to set limits. No doctor can fix everybody and a few patients with MUS also have severe personality disorders. GPs in particular sometimes feel a sense of failure if the doctor–patient relationship is not as good as they expect. If that is the case discuss it with a colleague and consider transferring the patient to the care of a different doctor. If all you are doing in consultations is maintaining the doctor–patient relationship you are not working effectively.

Setting safety nets

The idea of safety netting is well established in medical training and has already been mentioned in Chapter 3. Remember though that a small proportion of patients with apparent MUS have an unrecognised physical disease. It makes sense to review patients at appropriate intervals but at least as important as reviewing is looking out for – and using – new information. It is perfectly reasonable to include both expectation of recovery with a safety net. 'I expect this will settle over the next few weeks, but if it doesn't, or if X happens, then come back and see me'.

Bringing it all together

This chapter has outlined a set of principles for managing patient with MUS and illustrated these with examples of generic skills and techniques. These will be applied to specific contexts in Chapters 7 to 13, but for now are summarised in Figure 6.1.

Further reading

Gask L, Dowrick C, Salmon P, Peters S, Morriss R. Reattribution reconsidered: narrative review and reflections on an educational intervention for medically unexplained symptoms in primary care settings. *J Psychosom Res* 2011;**71**:325–34.

Burton C, Weller D, Worth A, Marsden W, Sharpe M. A primary care symptoms clinic for patients with medically unexplained symptoms: pilot randomised trial. *BMJOpen* 2012;**2**:e000513.

Woolfolk RL, Allen LA. *Treating Somatization: A Cognitive Behavioral Approach.* Guilford Press, New York, 2006.

CHAPTER 7

Palpitations, Chest Pain and Breathlessness

Chris Burton

University of Aberdeen, Aberdeen, UK

> **OVERVIEW**
>
> - Palpitations can be managed as a medically unexplained symptom by the GP where the clinical picture is very low risk or investigations show only sinus tachycardia
> - Chest pain, although a common medically unexplained symptom always warrants careful assessment
> - Breathlessness often has mixed physical and behavioural components – simple breathing control techniques are helpful for many patients
> - Palpitations, chest pain and breathlessness are commonly associated with anxiety and panic disorders. Consider these in patients with unexplained symptoms at any age

Introduction

Palpitations, chest pain and breathlessness are three common symptoms that patients present to GPs. All three are common medically unexplained symptoms (MUS) but all can be manifestations of life-threatening disease. Palpitations, chest pain and breathless are commonly associated with anxiety or panic and when assessed as low risk can be explained and managed as variations in autonomic function, often with secondary amplification. Although they commonly overlap, this chapter will deal with each of the three separately.

Palpitations

Epidemiology in primary care

Around 0.5% of patients consult a GP with some form of palpitations (awareness of possible abnormality of the heart beat) per year. Around one-third of these will have a detectable arrhythmia – although not all of these will be clinically important. The probability of significant arrhythmia increases with age.

GP assessment

The aim of GP assessment of new onset palpitations is to decide whether further investigation is warranted or whether the patient

should be managed as having innocent palpitations – a medically unexplained symptom. Investigation should include history, examination, electrocardiogram (ECG) and tests for anaemia and thyroid disorder.

Typical features of functional symptoms

Functional palpitations (either sinus tachycardia or heightened awareness of physiological variations in rhythm) may be reported as a fast heart rate, missed heartbeats or as pounding. Very brief (one or two beats) disturbances of rhythm or a regular rate less than 100, particularly if associated with a sense of pounding are strong pointers to functional symptoms.

> **Scenario 1**
>
> *'John' is a 28-year-old factory worker who regularly works out. He has noticed that sometimes when at home his heart pounds. It never occurs at work or in the gym and he tends to notice it especially when he's falling asleep. He demonstrates a regular heart rate during episodes of 80/min and recognises the feeling of his heart pounding out of his chest.*

Typical features of organic symptoms and red flag symptoms

In many cases the history and examination between episodes are of little value in differentiating organic tachycardia from innocent palpitation. Table 7.1 lists the likelihood ratios for various features as predictors of organic tachycardia. Although no feature on its own is sufficiently predictive, co-occurrence of several (for instance short episodes of pounding that do not occur during sleep or at work) strongly suggests a functional cause.

Palpitations associated with exercise, and with collapse are both alarm symptoms (for cardiomyopathy and ventricular arrhythmias in particular) as is palpitation associated with typical ischaemic chest pain. Any of these features should lead to referral, possibly urgently.

History and examination tips

The ideal is to examine the patient, and obtain an ECG, when they have their symptoms but this is usually not possible. If, during the

ABC of Medically Unexplained Symptoms, First Edition.
Edited by Christopher Burton.
© 2013 John Wiley & Sons, Ltd. Published 2013 by John Wiley & Sons, Ltd.

Table 7.1 Probability of arrythymia associated with clinical features in patients with palpitation.

Characteristic of palpitations	Likelihood ratio for arrhythmia
Epidemiology	
Presence of cardiac disease	2.0
Panic disorder	0.3
History	
Palpitations during sleep (not before sleep)	2.3
Palpitations at work	2.2
Palpitations lasting <5 min	0.4
Pounding sensation in chest	0.1
Examination	
Visible neck pulsation	2.7

Interpreting likelihood ratios: likelihood ratio >1 indicates increased probability of organic tachycardia; likelihood ratio <1 indicates reduced probability.

consultation, the patient suddenly appears concerned it is worth asking if their symptoms are present and checking the pulse. When taking the pulse, if you notice a missed beat, then ask the patient if they noticed it – increased awareness of minor variants such as ectopics is associated with anxiety disorders. If the pulse is normal then get the patient to tap out their abnormal rhythm and check whether it was regular – 'could you tap your foot to it?' If in doubt it can help to demonstrate a regular rhythm at 90 beats/min, and at 150 and an irregular rhythm to give the patient a choice.

Even though you know it will probably be normal, you should examine the heart properly. Emphasise to the patient that you are being thorough. Arrange an ECG, either within the consultation or in the near future and a clear plan for review. Arrange blood tests for anaemia and thyroid function, explaining that you expect them to be normal but are checking in order to be thorough.

It is worth considering anxiety (or less likely depression) in association with palpitations. Ask about sleep and concentration, listen for other symptoms commonly associated with anxiety or for patient-volunteered concerns.

Clinical decision

By the time you have completed the history and examination you should be able to classify the patient as having either low or increased probability of tachycardia.

Referral and Investigations

Patients with very low risk (episodes lasting less than 5 min, strong pounding, not occurring at work or when asleep) do not usually warrant further investigation. There is some evidence that a normal ambulatory ECG monitoring test *does not* increase reassurance.

Other patients warrant some form of continuous or episodic monitoring. Explain when referring patients that tachycardias are often physiological and that the test may show normal variations in heart rate with no sign of disease.

Explanation
Low probability of palpitations

The key aim of explanation is to normalise the potentially threatening symptom. Three component mechanisms are appropriate here:

normal ectopic beats; variable autonomic control and symptom awareness.

Normal ectopic beats warrant a simple but clear explanation (Box 7.1).

> Box 7.1 **Ectopic beats**
>
> *Everyone's heart sometimes has extra or missing heart beats. They are not a sign of disease. Usually we don't notice them but sometimes the brain gets tuned into these minor variations and notices them. That 'noticing' sometimes leads to 'looking out for' and so you can end up being aware of every change, even the normal ones.*
>
> *Now you know these extra beats are normal, it is safe to ignore them. You may need to practice reminding yourself that they are normal and harmless for a while until this becomes second nature.*

The variable autonomic control explanation accepts that the heart rate is continually changing under 'autopilot' control. Sometimes when resting, there are short bursts of unexpected activity. The key point is that when the system needs to respond it does so (everything is healthy, it works fine when exercising) but sometimes when resting or settling down at night, there are noticeable changes.

Symptom awareness links to variable autonomic control by amplifying the unexpected (but normal) changes in heart rate at rest. It makes sense that if something unexpected happens then the body will keep an eye out to see if it happens again. Sometimes this leads to a vicious circle of amplification and awareness (see Chapters 1 and 15).

Normal ambulatory ECG/event monitoring

Assuming the patient had symptoms associated with no rhythm disturbance then it is important to rationalise the patient's genuine awareness of the heartbeat and not imply that they were imagining it. This explanation will probably involve elements of variable autonomic control and symptom awareness as described above.

Specific treatment

Patients with disruptive but harmless awareness of their heartbeat may benefit from a low-dose beta-blocker. There have been only a few small studies in specialist care of brief cognitive-behavioural interventions for patients with palpitations, these suggest benefit but do not provide definitive evidence.

Chest pain

This section addresses two particular problems with chest pain: assessment of new chest pain and management of patients with angina-like pain after normal cardiac investigations.

Epidemiology in primary care

Chest pain symptoms are relatively common in primary care (lifetime incidence 20–40%, annual incidence around 1%).

Although many cases are either obviously due to disease – most commonly coronary heart disease (CHD) or oesophageal reflux – many are not. Observational studies suggest that around 5% of patients with undifferentiated chest pain (no clear diagnosis within 2 weeks) are subsequently found to have heart disease: thus, some patients initially thought to have medically unexplained chest pain do have, or develop, heart disease. A smaller number also turn out to have cancer or another serious illness. Even when initial assessment confers low risk, it is important for the GP to watch for changes in the clinical picture that point to disease.

GP assessment of new chest pain

The aim of the GP assessment of chest pain should be to assess the probability of cardiac or pulmonary disease and plan management accordingly. Low-risk chest pain tends to be either intense but very transient, lasting only a few seconds, or persistent over several days with little variation. In contrast to stable ischaemic pain it has no consistent relationship to effort or rest.

Table 7.2 shows a recently validated risk score for use in primary care for new patients presenting with chest pain. Using a cut-off score of three or more out of five it has a sensitivity of 86% and specificity of 75% for coronary heart disease.

History and examination tips

Take your time with a chest pain history. Listen while the patient describes the pain. Ask what it *feels* like – and leave the patient room to answer: you might get a description such as 'sharp', a simile ('like a knife going in)', an attribution ('I think it might be my heart') or an emotional response ('It's worrying'). These latter responses are particularly important in view of the patient attribution question in Table 7.2. Ask about relationship to exercise, breathing and rest. If necessary be specific: 'of the last 10 times it's come on, how many times were you sitting at home'.

In patients with chest pain you need to examine the heart. Although this is unlikely to yield information (although symptomatic aortic stenosis needs urgent referral) it is necessary and demonstrates that you are being thorough. It also means you can test for palpation tenderness (Table 7.2). In low-risk patients explain

Table 7.2 Score for risk of heart disease in primary care patients with chest pain.

Characteristic of chest pain	Points
Epidemiology	
Male aged ≥55 or female ≥65	1
Any prior clinical vascular disease (coronary, peripheral or cerebrovascular)	1
History	
Worse during exercise	1
Patient 'concerned that the pain is cardiac' or 'feeling very concerned about the pain'	1
Examination	
Pain *not* reproduced by palpation	1

Total score: ≥3 probability of coronary heart disease (CHD) at least 33%; ≤2 probability of CHD <3%.

that you have listened carefully to the heart and that it sounds OK (don't say this if you suspect disease, you may promote false reassurance).

Scenario 2

'Alex' is a 34-year-old mechanic. He reports pain in his chest over the last 4 weeks that has occasionally come on after exercise but has mostly occurred sitting at home or in the car. On closer questioning the pain has never occurred during manual effort or exercise, he feels the pain might represent an early sign of heart disease as his father was affected (in his 60s); pressure over the left parasternal area reproduces his discomfort.

Investigations and referral

Most hospitals have specific guidelines about whom to refer for chest pain assessment. Apart from some simple things like lipids etc the decisions about investigation are going to be made by specialists so they will follow from referral. If the pain sounds at all suspicious of pleural, rib or spine disease, remember to think of full blood count (FBC), c-reactive protein (CRP) and chest x-ray.

If investigating or referring patients who are not obviously at high risk of CHD, it is worth telling them in advance that the results of the tests may well be negative. Explain that some patients have pain that sounds like angina but is not due to heart disease; that this is common, and that it is not generally serious. Offer to see the patient after they have been for investigation. A small number of trials have shown that when patients receive information before tests that offers acceptable mechanisms for negative results this is associated with greater reassurance.

Explanation

Remember that successful reassurance needs two components: why the patient does not have a serious condition and why (probably) their current symptom is happening.

Low-risk patients

For low-risk patients whom you manage yourself, first restate why the pain does not have characteristics of heart pain. Use the tenderness and exercise features of the five-item score: for instance explain that if there is tenderness then the pain is coming from the muscles or costochondal joints, and that the heart is too well protected to allow pressure to hurt it. Consider using an analogy:

The heart is your body's motor, if there's something wrong with it then it will give you problems when you are making it work harder. But it seems that when you are busy and active it actually works fine – that's a very good sign.

Sometimes there are sufficient clinical grounds to explain the pain as due to a specific problem – for instance costochondral pain or reflux. If there are not, it is reasonable to accept that pain 'from the chest but not from the heart' like this is fairly common and tends to settle. The key point is that as the pain has been medically assessed as low risk, it is safe for the patient to *not* keep checking it and to try to ignore it. If the patient remains concerned – and you remain sure this is a low-risk situation – consider panic, anxiety or depression; all of these are fairly common (>10%) in patients attending secondary care with chest pain. A symptom amplification explanation can help to rationalise intrusive symptoms.

> *Your body uses symptoms to protect you: to warn that something might be wrong. In the case of something important like your heart it will often keep doing that, even if it's a false alarm. This makes it difficult for you to ignore. However, when you are busy – even though you are working your heart harder – you don't notice it. So, if you have been busy and it was fine and then it comes on when you are resting, it is safe to distract yourself from the discomfort.*

Explanation after negative cardiac investigations

Some patients will have investigations that effectively rule out significant coronary disease. Coronary angiography, coronary computed tomography (CT) and radionuclide scan may all do this but it is important to recognise that exercise ECG is much less effective in ruling out disease. The exact cause of pain in chest pain with normal coronary arteries remains contentious – most patients probably have a mix of dysfunctional small vessel perfusion and heightened awareness.

A recent Cochrane systematic review showed modest to moderate benefit from structured psychological interventions (mostly cognitive behavioural) in patients with chest pain and normal coronary arteries. These were relatively intensive interventions and the role for most GPs in managing these patients may be to refer to, and encourage attendance at, any available programme.

Specific treatment

Some patients with chest pain but normal coronary arteries will find benefit from beta-blockers, calcium channel blockers or nitrates. Depending on cardiologist opinion you might use these, but remember they are for symptom control, not proof that there actually is disease present.

Breathlessness

Epidemiology in primary care

Breathlessness is a relatively uncommon cause for attending the GP in the absence of respiratory disease but a substantial proportion of patients with lung conditions have superadded dysfunctional breathing. In addition, a few patients will present each year with acute hyperventilation associated with panic attacks.

On the other hand, a perception of breathlessness is common among patients with MUS and shortness of breath is one of the items on the PHQ15 screening tool. It is also a common cause of limited capacity in patients with multiple MUS.

GP assessment

GPs should consider dysfunctional breathing in patients where breathlessness is at odds with clinical findings – this may be in the case of asthma or chronic obstructive pulmonary disease (COPD) where symptoms seem disproportionate to signs and lung function – or it may occur along with non-cardiac chest pain. However, it is important to remember that some organic causes of breathlessness (especially pulmonary embolism) can present with with intense breathlessness and few objective signs other than distress. This may result in a life-threatening condition being misdiagnosis as functional hyperventilation.

Typical features of functional symptoms

Table 7.3 lists a number of items associated with dysfunctional breathing and included in the Nijmegen Hyperventilation Questionnaire. The value of the questionnaire in routine care is still uncertain and for many patients the pattern of breathing (typically hyper-inflated with use of chest and accessory muscles) may be a more important phenomenon than changes in CO_2.

Functional breathlessness is commonly associated with light-headedness and alarm but less often with pins and needles. Carpo-pedal spasm is rare and its absence does not rule out hyperventilation/dysfunctional breathing.

Examination tips

Listen for any unusual breathing patterns while the patient is telling you their history. Stopping for breath, or unusual breaths or sighs, during speech should make you suspicious. Look for the patient becoming uncomfortable or short of breath as you listen to their chest – if in doubt have them take a few more deep breaths or have them take 20 deep breaths 'as if you've just gone upstairs quickly'. Breathlessness brought on by deeper breathing is likely to indicate dysfunctional breathing.

Explanation

There are two key elements to explanation, first reassuring that the breathlessness is not caused by lung disease and second explaining why it is happening.

In addition to feeding back normal findings (breath sounds, spirometry), if your examination provoked symptoms, point out that disease-related breathlessness occurs when there is not enough oxygen getting into the body. However, during the examination the patient had deliberately breathed more deeply than usual so there was more than enough oxygen.

It is sometimes useful to explain about hyperventilation – where breathing too much lowers the level of CO_2 – however, although this is a reasonable argument there is no easy way of demonstrating it. In contrast it is simple to demonstrate dysfunctional breathing (Box 7.2).

Table 7.3 Typical features associated with hyperventilation.

Respiratory	Additional
Fast or deep breathing	Tightness around the mouth
Difficulty in taking a deep breath	Dizziness
Tightness across the chest	Feeling distant or unreal
	Palpitations

Box 7.2 **Dysfunctional breathing**

When a person's body needs extra oxygen in an emergency there are extra muscles to inflate the lungs more than normal and move extra air in and out. Sometimes this system gets a false alarm and it makes the lungs too full. To see what it feels like, take a deep breath in, then a small breath out – now try and take another deep breath . . . you can't. Does this feel familiar? [it often will]. *Now breathe all the way out, like a balloon deflating* [show them yourself] *and then try and take a deep breath – see how much easier it is.*

When you go to do something that might make you breathless, or if you are a bit anxious about your breathing, you will tend to fill up your lungs with extra air just in case. This is completely normal and understandable, but it gets in the way. Instead, I want you to think what an athlete does – for instance a weightlifter or a long jumper – just before he starts. You'd think that he would take a big breath in [demonstrate] *wouldn't you. So what does he actually do? . . . . He breathes right out* [demonstrate]. *It seems wrong doesn't it, but they all do it. That's because if you start with empty lungs, you can easily fill them once you start, but if you start with them full, the moment you try to breathe in, you will find you can't.*

Conclusion

Palpitations, chest pain and breathlessness are common symptoms in primary care. GPs have a role both in assessing whether they are organic and in actively managing those with a functional component. All these symptoms are commonly associated with anxiety disorders and it is important to consider this in the assessment.

Further reading

Bosner S, Haasenritter J, Becker A, *et al.* 2010, Ruling out coronary artery disease in primary care: development and validation of a simple prediction rule. *CMAJ* 2010;**182**:1295–300.

Chan T, Worster A. Evidence-based emergency medicine. The clinical diagnosis of arrhythmias in patients presenting with palpitations. *Ann Emerg Med* 2011;**57**:303–4.

Courtney R, van Dixhoorn J, Greenwood KM, Anthonissen EL. Medically unexplained dyspnea: partly moderated by dysfunctional (thoracic dominant) breathing pattern. *J Asthma* 2011;**48**:259–65.

CHAPTER 8

Headache

David P. Kernick

St Thomas Medical Group, Exeter, UK

OVERVIEW

- Headache has a considerable impact upon the lives of sufferers but the condition is poorly managed
- The initial aim of the headache consultation is to exclude serious pathology
- Migraine is the most common headache presentation in primary care in both adults and children
- Analgesic-overuse headache is common and should not be overlooked
- An underlying brain tumour is a common concern for patient and GP. Only investigate if there is a sound clinical indication: investigation can cause more anxiety than it relieves

Introduction

Headache is one of the common symptoms presented in primary care. Like many other symptoms in this book it can represent either serious disease, a cause of long-term distress or be intermittent and self-limiting.

Epidemiology in primary care

Over a 3-month period, 70% of the adult population will experience headache. In total 4% of GP consultations are for headache and 4% of headache consultations will result in a referral to secondary care. Including school-age children, 20% of the population have headache that has an impact on their quality of life.

Of all headaches, 5% are secondary i.e. there is a demonstrable pathology (including infections such as influenza as well as serious disease) and 95% are primary i.e. there is no observable underlying pathology. Primary headache is classified according to its clinical presentation. Here the basis of the headache is probably at a molecular level although certain headache presentations can be identified with activity in specific areas of the brain. Migraine (annual prevalence 15% in females and 8% in males) and tension-type headache (annual prevalence 70%) are the most common primary headaches and the ones that show most varia-

tion in response to changing circumstances, including psychosocial stress. A full classification of headaches can be found at the International Headache Society (HIS) website: www.ihs-headache.org/).

Table 8.1 shows estimates of the incidence of some important headache presentations in primary care.

GP assessment

The aim of management for the practitioner is to exclude a secondary headache, diagnose the appropriate primary headache, reduce any factors modifying the primary headache and treat accordingly.

Typical features of functional symptoms

Tension-type headache

The mechanisms underlying tension-type headache are poorly understood. The headache is usually dull and bilateral, it is often occipital but may be fronto-temporal. It is the commonest cause of a headache that is present all day every day. Patients with tension-type headache will keep going, in contrast to those with migraine who will want to lie down in a quiet, darkened room. Tension-type headache often coexists with migraine and some argue that in many cases tension-type headache is part of the migraine spectrum and based on similar neural mechanisms.

Medication-overuse headache

Of all primary headaches 10% will be complicated by medication-overuse headache, which often presents diagnostic difficulties if

Table 8.1 Estimates of the incidence of some important headache presentations in primary care.

Diagnosis	Incidence[1] (%)
Migraine	73
Other primary headache (predominantly tension type)	23
Subarachnoid haemorrhage	0.05
Meningitis	0.02
Temporal arteritis	0.02
Primary tumour	0.09
Other secondary headache	3.8

[1]Up to 10% of primary headaches can be complicated by medication overuse headache.

ABC of Medically Unexplained Symptoms, First Edition.
Edited by Christopher Burton.
© 2013 John Wiley & Sons, Ltd. Published 2013 by John Wiley & Sons, Ltd.

not excluded. Medication overuse headache does not have specific clinical features, but should be suspected when headaches worsen in patients taking triptans or opioid containing analgesics on 10 or more days per month or paracetamol or NSAIDs on 15 or more days per month.

Typical features of organic symptoms

There are three types of headache to consider: headaches representing serious disease, migraine and the defined primary headache syndromes.

Headaches representing serious disease

It is essential when assessing patients with headache to consider serious causes. The main ones – but not all – are listed in Table 8.2 along with useful predictive features.

Brain tumours

A major concern for patients and doctors is that a headache presentation reflects an underlying tumour. Brain tumours are uncommon among patients with headache in primary care. Around three-quarters occur in patients aged over 50.

The probability of a brain tumour in three clinical situations is shown in Box 8.1. In each of these situations the risk of tumour is less than 1%.

> **Box 8.1 Risk of primary brain tumour in primary care**
>
> • Headache presentation to GP: 1 in 1000
> • Headache presentation to GP if migraine or tension-type headache can be diagnosed on clinical grounds: 1 in 2000

• Isolated headache where no clinical diagnosis can be made after 8 weeks: 1 in 120

Some clinical features are associated with increased risk of tumour or other intracranial pathology and when these are present, urgent investigation is indicated (Box 8.2)

> **Box 8.2 Symptoms and signs suggesting possibility of secondary headache**
>
> • Worsening headache with fever
> • Thunderclap headache
> • New-onset neurological deficit
> • New-onset cognitive dysfunction
> • Change in personality
> • Impaired level of consciousness
> • Head trauma within 3 months
> • Headache triggered by cough, vasalva or sneeze
> • Headache triggered by exercise
> • Headache that changes with posture
> • Clinical features of giant cell arteritis
> • Clinical features of glaucoma
> • Significant change in characteristics of headache
> • Atypical aura

Migraine

Migraine is the most common headache presentation in primary care. Although formal criteria are quite specific, from a clinical perspective they may be relaxed. Answering yes to two out of three simple questions effectively identifies migraine sufferers (Box 8.3)

Table 8.2 Predictive features of serious causes of headache.

Headache	Useful predictive features
Emergency	
Meningitis	No feature is invariably present The following are common: fever (85%), neck stiffness (70%), alteration in mental status (67%), jolt accentuation of headache (97%)
Subarachnoid haemorrhage	Consider if this is the patient's worst ever headache The most common presentation is a 'thunderclap headache' that reaches maximum intensity within 10 s and lasts for a few hours 12% of such patients have a subarachnoid haemorrhage rising to 25% if examination is abnormal Other features include occipital location, nausea, neck stiffness, impaired consciousness
Temporal arteritis	Always think of this in anyone over 50 The headache can mimic the features of other headaches Check inflammatory markers, although 5% are normal
Others	Malignant hypertension (diastolic >120 and papilloedema); carotid artery dissection (injury); venous sinus thrombosis (pregnancy/hypercoagulable)
Urgent	
Tumours	See main text
Carbon monoxide poisoning	Ask about headache in other family members and type of heating

Other primary headaches

Although not common, most primary care practices will have some patients with these. The less common primary headaches include cluster headache, paroxysmal hemicrania and other syndromes. They are typically unpleasant and disruptive. Adequate description of these headache syndromes is beyond the scope of this book but you must be aware of them. The IHS website section on primary headaches is an excellent resource.

History and examination tips

In addition to questions to check for red flag symptoms, there are six key questions for the headache patient, as outlined in Table 8.3.

The examination

Although the relationship between blood pressure and headache is contested, blood pressure and fundoscopy are minimum examinations at the first presentation. A quick neurological examination that will elicit the most likely pathological findings is shown in Table 8.4. If the history is strongly in keeping with tension-type headache, examine the neck and look for painful trigger areas. Although muscle tension probably does not actually cause the headache, increased sensitivity to, or awareness of, pain is common in tension-type headache and eliciting it allows you to include it in your explanation.

Clinical decision

Following a history and examination headache should be classified as secondary (or possibly secondary) or primary. Most secondary headaches will need either immediate or urgent management but in some cases a period of observation with careful follow-up is appropriate. Examples of this include headache following minor trauma, stable headache that has a significant pattern change, headache that awakes from sleep.

Where the diagnosis is unclear, if a primary headache diagnosis cannot be made at 6–8 weeks, you should consider referral or investigation. Imaging (CT/magnetic resonance imaging (MRI)) is usually able to detect tumours and is indicated for patients whose pre-test probability of tumour is greater than 1%.

Imaging does little to reassure patients with headache in the long term even when negative and finds unexpected abnormalities in 10% of investigations, which may lead to additional worry. In view of this you should not arrange imaging for reassurance alone.

Explanation

Aim to give positive reassurance, for instance using the terms 'tension-type headache' or 'medication-overuse headache'. Although tension-type headache probably is not actually caused by muscle tension, the label is sometimes sufficient for patients to raise their own concerns about psychosocial stress.

Specific treatment

Treatment of the specific headache syndromes is covered by numerous guidelines such as the British Association for Study of Headache. For tension-type headache, simple analgesics and NSAIDs can be helpful. In some cases a 3-week course of NSAID may be reasonable to reduce the pain burden. Beware, though of leading to long-term analgesic use and medication-overuse headache. Physiotherapy addressing cervical spine function and posture can be

Table 8.3 Key questions for a patient with headache.

Question	Rationale
How much and how often is the patient taking painkillers?	Often the presenting headache is complicated by superimposed medication-overuse headache and there can be no progress on management until excessive analgesic use is abolished
How many types of headache does the patient recognise?	Most migraine sufferers will recognise a number of different types of headache. Concentrate on the most problematic headache, the others will almost certainly be part of the migraine spectrum
What impact does the headache have when it is there?	Migraine sufferers want to lie down in a quiet, dark room Tension-type headache suffers will keep going Cluster headache sufferers will want to pace the room and bang their head against the wall
Is there a family history of troublesome headache?	If there is, then this points to migraine
What does the patient think (or worry) may be causing their headache?	If patients think they have migraine there is a high chance that they will be correct. Explore triggers. Patients may also offer concern about serious pathology or suggest stress, validate these concerns and include them in your explanation
Does the patient have an anxiety or depressive disorder	Both of these commonly occur along with migraine and tension-type headache. The direction of causality is unknown but migraine may share some common pathophysiological pathways

Table 8.4 The neurological examination.

While patient is standing	
Ask the patient to:	**Tests:**
Close your eyes and stand with your feet together (Romberg)	Midline cerebellar; dorsal column; proprioception
Open your eyes and walk heel to toe	Midline cerebellar; dorsal column; proprioception
Walk on your tiptoes	Power of dorsiflexion
Walk on your heels	Power of plantar flexion
Close your eyes and hold your hands out straight in front of you with your palms flat and facing upwards	Hemisphere lesions (e.g. left hemisphere lesion, right hand will bend in and drift up)
	Neglect (e.g. left parietal lesion, right hand will drop down)
Keep your eyes closed. Touch your nose with the fingertip that I touch (person testing uses their own finger to touch a couple of the patient's fingertips in turn)	Light touch and finger-nose test (cerebellar or sensory ataxia and light-touch in fingertip)
Open your eyes and with your arms outstretched, pretend to play the piano	Fine finger movements
	Pyramidal and extrapyramidal function
Tap the back of one hand with your other hand. Change hands and repeat	Ataxia
Screw your eyes up tight and then relax and open your eyes	Pupil dilation and constriction Horner's syndrome Lower motor neurone lesion
Bare your teeth/grin	Upper motor neurone facial weakness
Stick your tongue out and wiggle it	Bulbar and pseudobulbar palsy
Stare at my face and point at the fingers which move (person testing has arms out to the side with index finger pointing. Arms stop in an arc and index finger is wiggled on each side in turn or together)	Temporal field defects (important visual field defects always involve one or other temporal field) Inattention (parietal lobe lesion)
Keeping your head still, stare at my finger and follow it up and down with your eyes (person testing draws a wide 'H' in the air)	Eye movements (cranial nerves III, IV, VI) Nystagmus; saccadic (jerky) eye movements

While patient is lying down	
Examine:	**Tests:**
Limb reflexes	Upper motor neurone lesion (brisk) Peripheral nerve or nerve root lesion (absent)
Plantar response	Upper motor neurone lesion (Babinski/extensor response)
Abdominal reflexes	Spinal cord disease
Funduscopy	Raised intracranial pressure (papilloedema) Optic atrophy
Pulse and blood pressure	Hypertension
If indicated, examine the chest, palpate breasts and abdomen	Systemic disease, e.g. neoplasia

Source: Reproduced from MacGregor A, Frith A, *ABC of Headache* 2009 with permission from John Wiley & Sons, Ltd. Table based on data from Elrington G, How to do a neurological examination in five minutes or less, *Pulse*, October 2007 www.pulsetoday.co.uk.

of benefit (especially when delivered by a therapist with particular interest). Amitriptyline and other pain modifying drugs can be effective: for details see Chapter 17.

Further reading

Kernick D, Goadsby P. *Manual of Headache Care*. Oxford University Press, Oxford, 2008.

Boardman H, Thomas E, Croft PR, Millson DS. Epidemiology of headache in an English district. *Cephalalgia* 2003;**23**:129–37.

Elrington G. How to do a neurological examination in five minutes or less. *Pulse*, 2007, October. www.pulsetoday.co.uk

Latinovic R, Gulliford M, Ridsdale L. Headache and migraine in primary care: consultation, prescription and referral rates in a large population. *J Neurol Neurosurg Psychiatry* 2006;**77**:385–7.

Kernick D, Ahmed F, Bahra A, *et al.* Imaging patients with suspected brain tumour. Guidance for primary care. *Br J Gen Pract* 2008;**58**(557):880–5.

Kernick D, Stapley S, Goadsby P, Hamilton W. What happens to new onset headache presented to primary care? A case-cohort study using electronic primary care records. *Cephalalgia* 2008;**28**(11):1188–95.

The British Association for the Study of Headache (www.bash.org.uk). Contains UK headache management guidelines.

Exeter Headache Clinic website: www.exeterheadacheclinic.org.uk.

National Institute for Clinical Excellence, CG150, diagnosis and management of headache in young persons and adults, 2012.

CHAPTER 9

Gastrointestinal Symptoms: Functional Dyspepsia and Irritable Bowel Syndrome

Henriëtte E. van der Horst

General Practice Department, VU Medical Centre, Amsterdam, The Netherlands

---

OVERVIEW

- Both functional dyspepsia and irritable bowel syndrome (IBS) are very common in primary care and can generally be managed by the GP
- A careful assessment will enable the GP to sort out those patients in whom symptoms may originate from a physical disease, requiring further investigation and/or referral
- Addressing patients' worries and providing information on symptoms and their management is the cornerstone of the GP's treatment
- If psychological factors are an important issue (such as coping with stress or anxiety) cognitive-behavioural therapy (CBT), or some form of relaxation therapy may be helpful

---

Introduction

All gastrointestinal symptoms reflect either pain or disturbed function, and in most cases this is not associated with organic disease. The functional gastrointestinal disorders have been exhaustively classified by the Rome Foundation, resulting in diagnostic criteria for a large number of functional gastrointestinal syndromes as shown in Figure 9.1.

The Rome III classification is compatible with a biopsychosocial model of functional gastrointestinal disorders. This is backed up by research into links between the brain and the gut (the so-called 'brain–gut axis') alongside changes in immune function and bacterial flora. To date the Rome III criteria have not been validated in primary care, and although they provide a useful framework they are restrictive in that they require symptoms to have been present for more than 6 months, which is often not the case when patients first present in primary care.

Functional dyspepsia

Dyspepsia refers to the experience of pain or discomfort in the upper abdomen. It is often a chronic or relapsing symptom.

ABC of Medically Unexplained Symptoms, First Edition.
Edited by Christopher Burton.
© 2013 John Wiley & Sons, Ltd. Published 2013 by John Wiley & Sons, Ltd.

The Rome III criteria for dyspepsia state that symptoms must have been present for at least the past 3 months and must have started 6 month prior to diagnosis. A prerequisite for the diagnosis of functional dyspepsia, and all function gastrointestinal syndromes is that there is no evidence of an underlying structural disease that is likely to explain the symptoms.

Scenario 1

'Brian' is a 36-year-old bank employee suffering from intermittent stomach complaints, mainly a burning sensation in his upper abdomen, sometimes with nausea. Gastroscopy 18 months ago was normal, with no evidence of Helicobacter pylori. Until now the episodes only lasted a few weeks at the most, and he coped by using over-the-counter medications. The reason for visiting his GP is that the symptoms are getting worse and have been present for more than a month now. He has stayed at home for a few days last week, because the symptoms were too bothersome although he doesn't think recent pressure at work is responsible.

Epidemiology in primary care

Dyspepsia affects 20–40% of the people in the UK and accounts for 1.2–4% of all GP consultations. In about half of these consultations the final diagnosis is functional dyspepsia. Most people with dyspepsia do not visit their GP but try to alleviate their symptoms with over-the-counter medication. Depression, anxiety and distress occur more often in patients with functional dyspepsia compared with the general population, and this probably influences their healthcare-seeking behaviour. In most cases the dyspepsia will disappear with or without treatment within months.

GP assessment

The aim of the GP assessment of dyspepsia should be to consider organic disease including peptic ulcer disease, *H. pylori* infection, reflux disease and cancer and to minimise symptoms. When symptoms persist, and if investigations are negative, the GP should consider a formal diagnosis of functional dyspepsia.

Typical features of functional dyspepsia

There is no pattern of symptoms that reliably predicts functional dyspepsia. Symptoms can be described as any of early fullness;

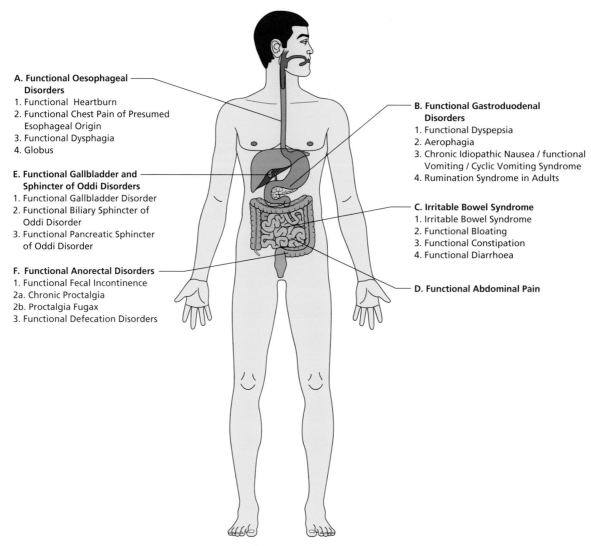

A. Functional Oesophageal Disorders
1. Functional Heartburn
2. Functional Chest Pain of Presumed Esophageal Origin
3. Functional Dysphagia
4. Globus

E. Functional Gallbladder and Sphincter of Oddi Disorders
1. Functional Gallbladder Disorder
2. Functional Biliary Sphincter of Oddi Disorder
3. Functional Pancreatic Sphincter of Oddi Disorder

F. Functional Anorectal Disorders
1. Functional Fecal Incontinence
2a. Chronic Proctalgia
2b. Proctalgia Fugax
3. Functional Defecation Disorders

B. Functional Gastroduodenal Disorders
1. Functional Dyspepsia
2. Aerophagia
3. Chronic Idiopathic Nausea / functional Vomiting / Cyclic Vomiting Syndrome
4. Rumination Syndrome in Adults

C. Irritable Bowel Syndrome
1. Irritable Bowel Syndrome
2. Functional Bloating
3. Functional Constipation
4. Functional Diarrhoea

D. Functional Abdominal Pain

Figure 9.1 Rome III functional gastrointestinal disorders.

bothersome postprandial fullness; epigastric pain; or epigastric burning, either alone or in combination. Bloating and belching (possibly secondary to air-swallowing) are suggestive but not diagnostic. IBS quite frequently co-occurs with functional dyspepsia and if this is present it may make functional dyspepsia more likely.

Typical features of organic disease

Around 50% of dyspepsia presenting to primary care is functional, which means the other 50% is not! There are several high-quality guidelines on the initial management of dyspepsia such as NICE CG17, which should be followed in the first instance.

History and examination tips

Ask about red flags: vomiting, weight loss, haematemesis, melena, and signs of blockage of food. Also ask for symptoms and a symptom pattern that points to an ulcer or a diaphragmatic hernia. and you should also check for other causes of dyspepsia including medicines (NSAIDs, anticoagulants, steroids, selective serotonin reuptake inhibitors (SSRIs) and over-the-counter medication) and alcohol.

Pay attention to the psychosocial dimensions. Is the patient particularly worried about the symptoms? Is there a possible explanation that has occurred to him? Do his symptoms have any social consequences such as missing any activities?

Although a physical examination rarely identifies positive findings in dyspepsia, it is an essential part of the consultation, indicating that you are taking the patient seriously. A negative investigation does not rule out pathology.

Investigations and referral

The appropriate investigation and management of dyspepsia of recent origin is well described in current guidelines. If the patient has persistent symptoms after a negative *H. pylori* test and endoscopy then you may need to consider alternative diagnoses. If there are no red flags, and the history is not typical of biliary colic, there is a risk that requesting an ultrasound 'just to be sure' may turn up asymptomatic gallstones, which are a common co-incidental finding and may lead to inappropriate surgery with poor outcome.

Explanation

Start by addressing any concerns that the patient has mentioned. Ensure that your explanation is in keeping with the patient's concerns and deal with these concerns by discussing with the patient why his symptoms do not indicate an underlying disease rather than dismissing it as an unnecessary worry. You can only effectively reassure the patients, if you have taken note of his concerns, and have done all the necessary tests (although this may be limited to a thorough history taking and physical examination).

After having addressed the patient's worries, explain that these symptoms are common, can be quite bothersome and in all probability do relate to a wide variety of factors. In quite a lot of people the intestines are overly sensitive to all kinds of stimuli such as food, smoking, hormonal changes, medication, stress etc. Both physiological and psychological factors may interact to produce symptoms.

If the patient's diet includes items that may contribute to the symptoms (fatty foods, alcohol, caffeine) consider reducing these to evaluate the effects. A food diary may be helpful to evaluate the relationship between symptoms and a particular substance. Smoking habits should be addressed because apart from all other consequences, smoking may contribute to dyspepsia symptoms.

Specific treatment

Prescribing an antacid for mild symptoms, or an H2 blocker or proton pump inhibitors (PPI) for more severe symptoms can relieve symptoms. Prescription should be for between 2 and 4 weeks, and then be evaluated. If psychological factors are an important issue (such as coping with stress or anxiety) CBT, or some form of relaxation therapy might be helpful if the patient is motivated for such a therapy. There is no need to persist with long term PPIs in patients with functional dyspepsia.

Scenario 1 (continued)

The GP examined Brian's abdomen and found no abnormality. She explained that sometime a healthy stomach just doesn't work properly and can lead to acid production or churning when it should be resting, then failing to work properly when it should be active. Given the previous normal tests and intermittent symptoms, she suggested that there were no danger signs here and that, with symptomatic treatment, the stomach would almost certainly settle down again and Brian was happy to wait for this. As Brian didn't think stress was bothering him, she didn't pursue that any further.

Irritable bowel syndrome

IBS is a fluctuating functional gastrointestinal disorder with a range of symptoms that may vary within an individual over time. Abdominal pain or discomfort and changes in bowel habit form the core of IBS, but symptoms can stem from the whole gastrointestinal system. Frequently, people with IBS also report non-gastrointestinal symptoms such as fatigue, urinary symptoms, headaches etc. Table 9.1 lists both the NICE and the ROME III diagnostic criteria for IBS.

Table 9.1 Clinical features of irritable bowel syndrome and diagnostic classifications.

Clinical feature	ROME III	NICE
Recurrent abdominal pain or discomfort At least 6 months since onset	✓	✓
AND ONE OF Pain improved with defecation Pain associated with change of stool form or frequency	✓	✓
WITH two or more of Altered stool passage (straining, urgency, incomplete evacuation) Abdominal bloating, distension, tension or hardness Symptoms made worse by eating Passage of mucus		✓
OPTIONAL symptoms that may support the diagnosis: lethargy; nausea; backache; bladder symptoms	✓	✓

NICE, National Institute for Health and Clinical Excellence.

As with functional dyspepsia, the guidelines for a formal diagnosis require the presence of symptoms for 6 months, however this does not have to be continuous: for instance, the Rome III criteria require several days per month in at least 3 of the 6 months. In terms of managing IBS it can be useful to think of three subtypes – whereas the current Rome III classification uses a single IBS category, previous versions described three subtypes – 'diarrhoea predominant', 'constipation predominant' or 'alternating symptom profiles'.

Epidemiology in primary care

IBS is very common, it affects about one in five people in the UK, although only a third of people suffering from the symptoms of IBS visit their doctor for these symptoms. It affects people of all ages and has the highest prevalence in the third and fourth decades. Prevalence is higher in women than in men.

IBS causes a lot of inconvenience for people, is associated with loss of work productivity and interferes with social activities in a substantial number of patients. The impact on quality of life is comparable with the impact of diseases such as diabetes and depression. In a subgroup of patients (about 10%) IBS follows a bacterial gastroenteritis and is usually the diarrhoea-predominant subtype. As in patients with functional dyspepsia, both depression and anxiety are more common among patients seeking healthcare for IBS, although this is probably a feature of healthcare seeking rather than IBS *per se*.

History and examination

Ask about the core symptoms of IBS, abdominal pain or discomfort, bloating and for additional symptoms such as constipation, diarrhoea, flatulence and dyspepsia. Also enquire about stool pattern and passing mucus with the stool. Symptoms like fatigue, nausea, backache and urinary symptoms often occur in patients with IBS. Enquire after a family history of inflammatory bowel disease (IBD) or colon cancer. In Table 9.2 the red flags for referral and risk factors are given.

Table 9.2 Red flags in possible irritable bowel syndrome.

History	Exam and Investigation
Rectal bleeding	Abdominal/rectal mass
Unintentional weight loss	Anaemia
A change in bowel habit to looser and/or more frequent stools persisting for more than 6 weeks (age over 60)	Raised inflammatory markers
Family history of bowel or ovarian cancer or of celiac disease	

Scenario 2

Claire' had an episode of gastroenteritis on holiday in Greece 2 years ago and following her return to the UK, she continued to have diarrhoea for 6 months during which time several tests were normal. Over the last few months her diarrhoea has returned along with bloating and urgency and she had become anxious about leaving the house in case she had to find a toilet. Examination was normal and the GP repeated Claire's FBC and inflammatory markers.

GP assessment

If alarm symptoms are absent and the symptoms and symptom pattern are compatible with IBS and the patient has had similar symptoms before, it is safe to make a diagnosis of IBS. If this is a first presentation you should consider investigations and if your history taking has elicited one or more red flags or if the physical examination has revealed an abnormality, this is mandatory.

Investigations and referral

Check FBC and inflammatory markers CRP or erythrocyte sedimentation rate (ESR). Remember that IBD can occur without raised inflammatory markers, so negative tests are insufficient to rule it out. If it has not already been carried out, order serological testing for coeliac disease. Some laboratories may offer faecal calprotectin testing – secondary care studies suggest that a negative result safely rules out IBD but this has not yet been evaluated in primary care. In women with new onset abdominal pain and bloating consider the possibility of ovarian carcinoma. Stool culture may be appropriate in patients with recent onset symptoms suggestive of diarrhoea predominant IBS.

Refer patients urgently if there are alarm symptoms and routinely if there is diagnostic uncertainty, or severe resistant symptoms. In the UK, GPs refer about one in seven cases to specialists.

Explanation

Start by addressing patient concerns or worries. Many people with IBS have concerns about a possible serious cause for their symptoms. Be willing to explain why you think their concern is unlikely rather than just dismissing it as an unnecessary worry. You can only effectively reassure the patients if you have taken note of their concerns and have done all the necessary tests as outlined above.

Explain that IBS is common, can be very bothersome and it is caused by multiple factors. In quite a lot of people the intestines are overly sensitive to all kinds of stimuli such as food, smoking, hormonal changes, medication, worry and stress and these may interact to produce symptoms. Recent research suggests that both severe gastrointestinal infections and prolonged stress may alter the brain–gut axis, resulting in normal stimuli being felt as abnormal.

Scenario 2 *(continued)*

Claire came back for her test results and was relieved to hear things were normal. She mentioned that a friend at work has Crohn's disease and has recently required major surgery. Her GP explained that sometimes a healthy bowel can go through spells of being sensitive and 'jumpy' and that this can sometimes leave people nervous about being in unfamiliar places in case they need to go to the toilet urgently. Claire then mentioned that during her Greek holiday she became ill on a bus and was terrified of being incontinent in public. Her GP acknowledged that was understandable and together they agreed that the chances of that happening now was pretty remote.

Most experts recommend that patients take regular meals and limit their intake of fatty foods, alcohol, caffeine and fizzy drinks. Some patient with constipation benefit from more dietary fibre, fruit and vegetables, but these can worsen symptoms for others. Physical exercise is not harmful and on the contrary might improve bowel function in patients with constipation. Some patients may exclude many food substances from their diet. Consider referral to a dietician for patients where simple advice seems insufficient.

Specific treatment
Pharmacological treatment

Bothersome predominant symptoms can sometimes be alleviated by medication. If pain is severe, consider offering antispasmodic agents, alongside dietary and lifestyle advice. Constipation in IBS usually responds to conventional bulking agents. Some patients find lactulose increases both pain and bloating. You should evaluate the effect in a month's time, if they do not report any improvement it is useless to go on with this therapy. For diarrhoea offer loperamide as the first choice, telling people how to adjust doses according to response, shown by stool consistency.

If symptom-focused medication has no effect on the pain and the patient wants to try further medication to alleviate symptoms then consider low dose amitriptyline 10–30 mg daily (see Chapter 17). You can try tricyclic antidepressants (TCAs) for their analgesic effect. Start at a low dose (5–10 mg equivalent of amitriptyline) taken once at night and review regularly, you may increase the dose but not exceed a daily dose of 30 mg.

Consider SSRIs only if TCAs are ineffective. If prescribing these drugs for the first time, follow-up after 4 weeks (monitor also the side effects to evaluate the benefits) and then every 6–12 months.

Psychological treatment

If psychological factors are an important issue (such as coping with stress or persisting anxiety) CBT, or some form of relaxation therapy might be helpful if the patient is motivated for such a therapy.

Also discuss referral for a psychological treatment with people whose symptoms do not respond to pharmacological treatments after 12 months and who develop a continuing symptom profile (refractory IBS). There is evidence for the effectiveness of CBT, both for individuals and groups, and for hypnotherapy.

Other functional gut syndromes

As Figure 9.1 shows, there are several other functional gut disorders that are not covered in this chapter. Most GPs will see a few patients with proctalgia fugax or levator ani syndrome in their professional career. Abdominal pain 'just like my gallbladder' after cholecystectomy is not uncommon and can be extremely distressing. Some patients have demonstrable Sphincter of Oddi spasm, others may have had IBS all along (and have had incidental gallstones treated). In some cases the problem appears to be a visceral pain disorder. The principles of managing these are similar to those for other conditions in this book.

Conclusion

The gastrointestinal system gives rise to many symptoms that are more often functional than pathological. Functional dyspepsia and IBS are the most common. Making use of the basic skills of history taking and physical examination the GP can safely establish a diagnosis of functional dyspepsia and IBS in the majority of cases. Providing reassurance and information on symptoms and their management will suffice in most patients. Symptomatic medication and/or psychological treatment are sometimes warranted.

Further reading

Drossman DA. The functional gastrointestinal disorders and the Rome III process. *Gastroenterol* 2006;**130**:1377–90.

National Institute for Health and Clinical Excellence. *Dyspepsia: Management of Dyspepsia in Adults in Primary Care*. NICE, London, 2004. Available at: http://guidance.nice.org.uk/CG17 (retrieved 27 July 2012).

National Institute for Health and Clinical Excellence. *Irritable Bowel Syndrome in Adults: Diagnosis and Management of Irritable Bowel Syndrome in Primary Care*. NICE, London, 2008. Available at: http://guidance.nice.org.uk/CG61 (retrieved 27 July 2012).

National Institute for Health and Clinical Excellence. *Coeliac Disease: Recognition and Assessment of Coeliac Disease*. NICE, London, 2009. Available at: http://guidance.nice.org.uk/CG86 (retrieved 27 July 2012).

Rome Foundation, The. *Rome III Diagnostic Criteria for Functional Gastrointestinal Disorders*. The Rome Foundation, Raleigh, NC, 2006. Available at: http://www.romecriteria.org/ (retrieved 28 July 2012).

CHAPTER 10

Pelvic and Reproductive System Symptoms

Nur Amalina Che Bakri[1], Camille Busby-Earle[2], Robby Steel[3] and Andrew W. Horne[1]

[1]MRC Centre for Reproductive Health, University of Edinburgh, Edinburgh, UK
[2]Simpson Centre for Reproductive Health, Royal Infirmary of Edinburgh, Edinburgh, UK
[3]Department of Psychological Medicine, Royal Infirmary of Edinburgh, Edinburgh, UK

OVERVIEW

- >50% of patients with chronic pelvic pain (CPP) have no obvious underlying pathology
- The diagnosis of functional CPP should be given as a positive statement not an expression of negative findings
- Central sensitisation plays an important part in CPP and needs to be explained carefully
- Vulvodynia and dyspareunia are commonly associated with CPP

Introduction

This chapter focuses on three common female pelvic symptoms: CPP, vulvodynia and dyspareunia. Although we categorise presentations as 'organic' or 'functional' it is important to recognise that these overlap: many women will have both organic pathology and functional symptoms.

Chronic pelvic pain

CPP is defined as an intermittent or constant pain in the lower abdomen or pelvis of at least 6 months' duration, not occurring exclusively with menstruation or intercourse and not associated with pregnancy, that causes functional disability or limits daily activities

Epidemiology in primary care

CPP affects 38 per 1000 women in general practice in the UK, which makes it as common as asthma or back pain. Patients with CPP make up approximately 20% of outpatient appointments in gynaecology clinics and cost the UK National Health Service (NHS) an estimated £158 million a year.

CPP can be associated with gynaecological conditions, such as endometriosis, and non-gynaecological conditions such as IBS, interstitial cystitis/bladder pain syndrome, musculoskeletal pain and fibromyalgia In more than 50% of patients, no cause for the painful symptoms can be found.

A history of abuse (physical, sexual and/or psychological) is more common in women with CPP.

GP assessment

The aim of GP assessment in women with CPP is to exclude pathological causes of CPP and to recognise patients with functional CPP. This can usually be achieved by taking a history and performing an examination so that only selected patients are referred to secondary care.

Typical features of organic symptoms

Endometriosis is found in 35–50% women with CPP. Cyclical pelvic pain (often associated with dysmenorrhoea and dyspareunia) in women of reproductive age is the most common symptom associated with the condition and merits referral to secondary care for investigation (see Box 10.1). The gold standard for diagnosing endometriosis is laparoscopy; there are no serum or urinary biomarkers of endometriosis. However, treatment of endometriosis, using drugs that cause ovarian suppression (e.g. combined oral contraceptive pill, progestogens, gonadotrophin-releasing hormone agonists), may be started prior to laparoscopy. If these drugs successfully alleviate symptoms, a laparoscopy is not always necessary.

Box 10.1 **Symptoms indicating possible endometriosis**

- Severe dysmenorrhoea
- Deep dyspareunia
- Chronic pelvic pain
- Ovulation pain
- Other cyclical or perimenstrual symptoms, e.g. bowel or bladder
- Infertility
- Dyschezia (pain on defaecation)

Adenomyosis is characterised by the same symptoms as endometriosis. It is more often diagnosed histologically following a hysterectomy but can be diagnosed by pelvic MRI. Adhesions due to previous surgery, pelvic infection or endometriosis are also associated with CPP but there is little evidence that division of adhesions reduces pelvic pain symptoms. Pelvic congestion

ABC of Medically Unexplained Symptoms, First Edition.
Edited by Christopher Burton.
© 2013 John Wiley & Sons, Ltd. Published 2013 by John Wiley & Sons, Ltd.

syndrome is the association of pelvic varicosities seen on MRI with pelvic pain. Ovarian suppression has been shown to be helpful.

Typical features of functional symptoms

Patients may use emotive language or employ dramatic metaphors when describing their symptoms (e.g. 'I feel as if I am being stabbed by a red-hot poker').

There may be inconsistencies in the presentation or history (e.g. the patient walks to the consulting room with normal gait and no apparent discomfort yet flinches with severe pain on superficial abdominal palpation). Such inconsistencies should not be interpreted as evidence of deception, they may reflect (subconscious) variations in the extent to which the patient is attending to the pain.

Patients with functional pelvic pain often present with other medically unexplained symptoms (MUS) and are often in contact with other hospital specialties (e.g. gastroenterology for IBS, rheumatology for fibromyalgia etc).

It is important to recognise that the presence of organic pathology does not exclude functional symptoms, indeed CPP is commonly preceded by physical disease. Although a history of abuse is a risk factor for CPP it is unlikely in a generalist consultation that you will identify this.

Scenario 1

'Sarah' is a 32-year-old office worker with a history of pelvic pain of 8 months duration. The pain is worse with menstruation and she takes regular non-steroidal analgesia to little effect. She has had to take time off her work due to the pain. She has previously been fit and well except for an admission with renal colic.

Her GP recognises the cyclic nature of her pain and discusses the possibility of endometriosis. She is keen to establish the diagnosis rather than treat symptomatically so her GP refers her for laparoscopy.

History and examination tips

The consultation process itself can be therapeutic. So in a consultation (or over a series of consultations) with a woman with CPP you should encourage the patient to describe her symptoms and the impact they have on her, including avoidance (work, recreation, sex) and allow her to express her worries (e.g. about cancer or infertility) and concerns. Where appropriate, enquire about a history of sexual and physical assault.

Abdominal palpation and internal pelvic examination should be performed – failure to perform an examination may be interpreted as evidence that you are not taking the symptoms seriously.

Investigation and referral

Endometriosis and pelvic adhesions can only be diagnosed by direct visualisation. Referral for a laparoscopy should therefore be considered in patients in whom there is a high suspicion of these conditions or concern about associated infertility.

If the history is suggestive of underlying pathology (see Box 10.1) or any abnormalities are found during examination, the woman should be referred for specialist assessment.

Explanations of functional CPP

Give the diagnosis as a positive statement, not as an expression of negative findings (e.g. 'You have chronic pelvic pain, this is a common condition, although we do not fully understand it'). Avoid terms such as 'psychological' or 'underlying depression' as a mechanism for pain. If patients persist in wanting a cause, consider using analogy. For example, most people will have experienced headache in their life and usually there will be no pathological explanation of this problem. Some patients may pick up on associations of headache and stress and extend this to pelvic pain inviting further discussion of psychosocial factors.

You might include the increased attention to symptoms that occurs when one is concerned or does not know what is going on. Consider framing the pain as 'safe but a nuisance' rather than a sign of danger. In terms of management, explain that although there is no specific treatment, you can work to reduce the symptoms and help the patient return to normal activities.

Scenario 1 *(continued)*

Sarah tells her GP that the gynaecologist just told her there was 'nothing sinister wrong'. Her GP recognises the annoyance in her voice: 'You seem a little upset about that. What are you thinking?'.

At this Sarah becomes tearful and asks what she is supposed to do about her pain. Exploring her understanding reveals that she sees no prospect of treatment: if a cause cannot be found, how can it be treated? She expresses her fear that 'something serious might have been missed'.

Sarah asks how she could possibly have pain without a cause. Her GP uses a previous episode of renal colic and its referred pain as a starting point for the idea that 'the body generates misleading pain signals'. After some discussion, Sarah accepts an explanation of 'pain fibres firing inappropriately' and welcomes this 'positive reassurance' (i.e. an explanation of what is causing her pain – as opposed to 'negative reassurance', which is a list of what isn't). She and the GP consider hormonal treatment with the combined oral contraceptive pill (COCP) but in the end agree to a trial of low-dose amitriptyline to 're-tune the pain signals'.

Specific management

After making a positive diagnosis of 'chronic pelvic pain', consider appropriate use of analgesic and additional drugs (see Chapter 17). Hormonal treatments can also be offered to help with cyclical pain (e.g. COCPs or – with specialist supervision – gonadotropin-releasing hormone (GnRH) agonists). Some patients will benefit from CBT – see Chapters 15 & 16. Some patients warrant specialist referral to liaison psychological services and pain teams: for instance if there are severe symptoms, marked impairment of function, risk of iatrogenic harm, or repeated cycles or referral.

Vulvodynia

Vulvodynia is defined as vulval discomfort, most often described as burning pain, occurring in the absence of relevant visible findings or a specific neurological disorder. Vulvodynia can either be provoked by pressure (vestibulodynia, previously called vulval vestibulitis) or unprovoked (dysaesthetic or essential vulvodynia). Both forms can be either localised (typically at the entrance to the vagina between 4 and 8 o'clock) or generalised.

Epidemiology in primary care

Localised vulvodynia is the most common cause of vulval pain: it commonly also causes dyspareunia in patients under the age of 50. It is characterised by typical historical clues e.g. pain is elicited on contact or after sexual intercourse or when using tampons. The incidence and prevalence of vulvodynia in the general practice setting in the UK is unknown.

GP assessment

The diagnosis of vulvodynia is clinical. The aim of GP assessment is to exclude pathological causes of vulval pain and to recognise patients with the condition. This can usually be achieved by taking a history and performing an examination. In most cases, vulvodynia can be managed by recommending simple health measures so that only selected patients require referral to secondary care.

Typical features of organic symptoms

Vulvovaginal candidiasis should always be suspected as a cause of vulval pain. Candidiasis is a very common infection affecting 75% of all women at some point in their lifetime and is associated with itch, erythema and often a white 'like a curd cheese' discharge. Herpes simplex and herpes zoster infection can be mistaken for vulvodynia as they can present without visible lesions. Patients will usually report previous episodes.

Fissures due to trauma at sexual intercourse can lead to vulval pain. Patients often describe the pain as like a 'papercut'. Contact allergic dermatitis and irritant dermatitis can usually be elicited from the history (e.g. overenthusiastic vulval hygiene). Lichen sclerosus and lichen planus have typical appearances but, where the diagnosis is in doubt referral is appropriate. Vulval carcinoma should be considered if there is persistent irritation, erosion and ulceration in addition to the vulval pain. Patients with these should be referred urgently.

Typical features of functional symptoms

Table 10.1 shows the characteristics of the provoked and unprovoked patterns of vulvodynia.

History, examination and investigation

The principles of history and examination of vulvodynia are very similar to those described for pelvic pain (above) with two additional features. You should also examine the mouth, perineum and

Table 10.1 Symptoms and signs of provoked and dysaesthetic vulvodynia.

Provoked vulvodynia (vestibulodynia)	Dysaesthetic (or essential) vulvodynia
Pain on contact e.g. coitus or tampon use; few symptoms when unprovoked	Spontaneous pain
Can be generalised around the vulva or localised	Pain is more diffuse and there is less dyspareunia
Most patients are pre-menopausal and sexually active	Peri- or post-menopausal women are usually affected
May be complicated by vaginismus	Urethral (pain, frequency) or anal symptoms common

perianal area as well as the vulva; these are all normal in vulvodynia. You can also conduct the Q-tip test (using a cotton swab) to test for pain on light pressure at different points around the vulva in a clockwise fashion. At each point ask the patient to quantify the pain, if any, from a scale of 0 to 10.

A vaginal swab should be obtained for microscopy and culture if infection is suspected.

Explanations and management

This follows similar patterns to CPP and uses a multifaceted approach to address local factors, central pain sensitivity and, if appropriate, psychological issues. This may require specialist skills.

Dyspareunia

Dyspareunia is defined as pain during or after sexual intercourse, which can be deep or superficial.

Epidemiology in primary care

It is difficult to estimate the incidence of dyspareunia as the majority of cases are not reported, however, it seems likely that between 10 and 20% of women are affected by dyspareunia at some point in their lives.

GP assessment

Dyspareunia commonly accompanies, or has features of CPP or vulvodynia and in many ways the assessment is similar to those other conditions. It involves considering physical (including structural change following surgery or childbirth), pathological and functional processes.

It is useful to classify dyspareunia as either superficial or deep and to determine whether pain is accompanied by vaginisimus – a tightness that prevents penetration. As with the other symptoms in this chapter, a careful explanation, with appropriate interpretation of the findings is important. It is important that this examination includes checking for cervical excitation tenderness and any pelvic mass.

Where appropriate, vaginal swabs taken should be sent for testing for candida, chlamydia and gonorrhoea. A mid-stream urine specimen should be collected to check for urinary tract infection.

In obtaining a sexual history, ask about libido, foreplay and non-penetrative sexual behaviour (and whether artificial lubricants have been useful). Involvement of the partner in the consultation can be helpful, they can bring insights and are likely to be involved in the management plan. However, it is important to ensure women have the opportunity to ask questions and/or make disclosures without their partner being present.

Explanation after a negative investigation

Explaining the condition, allaying any fears and reassuring the patient that the condition is not infectious or related to cancer is essential. Providing women with patient information sheets is often helpful.

Specific management

This may need referral to a sex therapist or specialist physiotherapist able to teach pelvic muscle control for vaginismus. In patients with a structural cause, Fenton's operation may be appropriate.

Other pelvic and reproductive symptoms

Bladder Pain Syndrome is the current preferred term for urinary symptoms with negative investigations although the term interstitial cystitis is still in widespread use. It commonly overlaps with CPP, vulvodynia and IBS and like them it appears to have a central pain sensitisation component. Men with persistent testicular pain are often labelled as having chronic epididymitis but this syndrome may be analogous to CPP in women.

Further reading

Damsted-Petersen C, Boyer SC, Pukall CF. Current perspectives in vulvodynia. *Womens Health* 2009;**5**(4):423–36.

Daniels JP, Khan KS. Chronic Pelvic Pain in Women. *BMJ* 2010;**341**:c4834.

Lotery HE, McClure N, Galask RP. Vulvodynia. *Lancet* 2004;**363**(9414): 1058–60.

Reed BD. Vulvodynia: diagnosis and management. *Am Fam Physician* 2006;**73**(7):1231–8.

Royal College of Obstetricians and Gynaecologists. *The Initial Management of Chronic Pelvic Pain (Green Top Guideline No 41)*. RCOG, London, 2012. Available at: http://www.rcog.org.uk/files/rcog-corp/CPP_GTG2ndEdition230512.pdf (retrieved 28 July 2012).

Royal College of Obstetricians and Gynaecologists. *The Investigation and Management of Endometriosis (Green Top Guideline No 24)*. RCOG, London, 2008. Available at: http://www.rcog.org.uk/files/rcog-corp/GTG2410022011.pdf (retrieved 28 July 2012).

Steege JF, Zolnoun DA. Evaluation and treatment of dyspareunia. *Obstet Gynecol* 2009;**113**(5):1124–36.

www.crh.ed.ac.uk/pelvicpain – pelvic pain website

www.endometriosis-uk.org – Endometriosis UK

www.nhs.uk/conditions/Vaginismus/Pages/Introduction.aspx – vaginismus

www.pelvicpain.org.uk – Pelvic Pain Support Network

www.vulvalpainsociety.org: Vulval Pain Society

CHAPTER 11

Widespread Musculoskeletal Pain

Barbara Nicholl, John McBeth and Christian Mallen

Arthritis Research UK Primary Care Centre, Keele University, Keele, UK

OVERVIEW

- Widespread pain involves multisite body pain often with symptoms in other body systems. It includes the syndrome of fibromyalgia
- Patients with widespread pain often have associated sleep and concentration difficulty that compound the impact of pain
- Explanations should include the idea of central pain and assure the patient that pain does not indicate damage or harm
- Optimal management varies from patient to patient, it may include non-pharmacological as well as pharmacological approaches

Introduction

Pain reported in multiple body sites is common. The term 'widespread pain' (which includes fibromyalgia) is used to describe pain that is present in left and right sides of the body and above and below the waist. The syndrome fibromyalgia is a more severe form of chronic widespread pain, in which patients also have additional somatic symptoms that have an impact on their functioning. In this chapter, we refer to widespread pain, but all points are applicable to fibromyalgia.

Epidemiology in primary care

Widespread pain and fibromyalgia are not discrete disorders that can be easily separated from normal experience. Widespread pain is common: approximately 11% of the general population have symptoms whereas 2% have fibromyalgia. Symptoms are more frequently reported by women. Both widespread pain and fibromyalgia are more common with increasing age (until approximately the sixth decade) and at all ages symptoms are associated with poor mental health and reduced health-related quality of life. It is unclear why the prevalence of widespread pain decreases in the oldest old, however, changes in risk factors (psychological symptoms and work factors) and altered pain processing are possible explanations.

ABC of Medically Unexplained Symptoms, First Edition.
Edited by Christopher Burton.
© 2013 John Wiley & Sons, Ltd. Published 2013 by John Wiley & Sons, Ltd.

Several causal mechanisms have been identified in patients with widespread pain. These include, central pain processing, stress response, and genetic, psychosocial and work factors; however, the extent to which widespread pain symptoms can be attributed to a specific organic cause is limited.

Typical features of functional symptoms

Widespread pain is defined as pain in the axial skeleton and at least two quadrants of the body with pain on both right and left sides and above and below the waist. Chronic widespread pain requires symptoms to have been present for at least 3 months.

Most patients with widespread pain also experience other physical symptoms. They frequently present with other symptoms indicative of IBS and fatigue. Some patients with widespread pain are recognisable as frequent attenders and individuals with widespread pain have a poorer outcome than those with regional pain, which indicates the usefulness of asking about pain elsewhere in the body when a patient consults with regional pain. Body manikins or the Widespread Pain Index can be used to assess how widespread an individual's pain is. Patients commonly have some degree of cognitive, mood and sleep problems; all of which should be taken into consideration when making decisions about clinical care, see Box 11.1.

Box 11.1 **Common non-pain presenting symptoms of a widespread pain disorder**

- Fatigue
- Sleep problems
- Irritable bowel
- Headaches
- Blurred vision
- Mood problems (particularly depressive and anxiety symptoms)
- Cognitive problems (e.g. difficulty concentrating)
- Weakness
- Overall functioning problems (e.g. inability to conduct usual activities and regular or prolonged time off work for symptoms)

Typical features of organic symptoms

Widespread pain can be associated with serious disease including inflammatory arthropathies, connective tissue diseases and a range

Table 11.1 Red flags suggesting serious disease in assessment of widespread pain.

History	Exam	Investigations
Fever/sweats	Synovitis	Anaemia
Unexplained weight loss	Tender MCP/MTP joints	Raised CRP/ESR
Morning joint stiffness	Lymphadenopathy	Abnormal urinalysis
New onset Raynaud's	Rash	
Visual disturbance	Neuromuscular signs	
Dry eyes and mouth		

CRP, C-reactive protein; ESR, Erythrocyte sedimentation rate; MCP, metacarpophalangeal joints; MTP, metatarsophalangeal.

of cancers. Morning joint stiffness lasting more than 30 min, weight loss or any of the other clinical features listed in Table 11.1 should alert you to the possibility of a serious cause.

History and examination tips

A structured history should include current symptom, previous musculoskeletal pain and other somatic symptoms, the evolution of the problem (is it acute or chronic?) and any involvement of other systems. Consider getting the patient to complete the Widespread Pain Index or the Fibromyalgia Symptom Scale in order to get a standardised measure of severity.

The examination has two roles: to exclude other disorders and to demonstrate empathy to the patient and give them confidence that their problem is being taken seriously. A tender point examination and count is no longer required for a fibromyalgia diagnosis. A structured musculoskeletal examination, such as the GALS (gait, arms, legs, spine) screening examination, which is taught by UK undergraduate medical schools, and is published in detail in Arthritis Research UK's student handbook (and accompanying DVD) on 'Clinical Assessment of the Musculoskeletal System', is a quick and useful way to assess the musculoskeletal system and exclude red flags. Further site-specific examinations should be carried out for any abnormalities observed. In addition to musculoskeletal examinations, a patient should be examined for other factors that may relate to a differential diagnosis, including those of concern that arose in the patient's history and examining for skin rashes, psoriasis and signs of neurological problems.

Investigations

A complete medical history and examination will help to determine what further investigations may be required. Box 11.2 lists recommended investigations for excluding other potential diagnostic explanations for the presenting pain.

Unless there is good clinical suspicion, vitamin D levels, rheumatoid factor and antinuclear antibody levels need not be tested. A small minority of patients may require referral for further investigations, as the clinician deems appropriate.

Explanation

Explanations of a widespread pain disorder should acknowledge the patient's pain, empathise with the impact that it has on their

---

Box 11.2 Recommended investigations in suspected widespread pain disorder

- Full blood count
- Erythrocyte sedimentation rate
- C-reactive protein
- Creatine kinase
- Calcium
- Alkaline phosphatise
- Blood glucose
- Thyroid-stimulating hormone
- Urinalysis for protein, blood and glucose

---

daily life and should be both realistic and reassure the patient that their symptoms are manageable.

Some patients will believe that their pain was brought on by an event such as a road traffic accident or a major emotional problem, such as the death of a spouse. Rather than contest this, consider using the idea of the event as a trigger, which resulted in a set of processes that are now keeping the problem going (see Chapters 15–16).

It is important to include in any explanation that there is no specific damage to muscles, bones or joints and therefore maintaining or regaining physical function is important and attainable, although consideration should be given to what other health problems the individual may have. It may also be useful to highlight that although widespread pain is not a psychological disorder, talking therapies may be useful to manage pain. Despite the patient having no obvious physical damage causing their pain, this does not make the pain any less real for the patient to cope with or the clinician to manage. A useful explanation is suggested in Box 11.3.

Box 11.3 Useful explanation for widespread pain

Widespread pain is a central pain processing problem. This means that the brain sometimes gets overloaded with pain signals that just won't stop. Nobody knows exactly why this happens but it seems that in widespread pain it is difficult for your body to switch some nerves off. The pain isn't a sign of damage to your bones, joints or muscles so maintaining (or regaining) physical activity is helpful and pain doesn't mean you are doing harm. There are treatments that can be used to change the way your body handles pain: these can reduce the pain and help you control it better.

Specific management

Patients should be reassured by their clinician that their pain symptoms can be managed and a good quality of life can be attained through a number of options that they may find beneficial. It is important to be realistic with the patient that it may take time to find the management plan that works best for them, however, maintaining positivity in managing patients with widespread pain is essential. Successful management requires a multidisciplinary approach, which addresses not only the pain symptoms but the other comorbid problems that the patient may have. Management approaches can be split into the following three areas.

Reassurance

Promoting the patient's own self-management of their symptoms through advice and written/online resources (see Box 11.4 for potential resources). Enabling a patient to cope with their widespread pain and to regain control of their life is vital.

Box 11.4 **Patient information sources about widespread pain**

The Pain Toolkit – information booklet to help people with persistent pain. Available online (www.paintoolkit.org/).

Arthritis Research UK patient information booklet: What is fibromyalgia? Available online or in print from Arthritis Research UK (www.arthritisresearchuk.org/~/media/Files/Arthritis-information /Conditions/2013-Fibromyalgia.ashx).

BMJ patient information: Fibromyalgia summary. Available online (http://bestpractice.bmj.com/best-practice/pdf/patient-summaries /en-gb/532236.pdf).

Arthritis Research UK self-help and daily living booklet: *Keep Moving*. Available online or in print from Arthritis Research UK (www.arthritisresearchuk.org/~/media/Files/Arthritis-information /Living-with-arthritis/2282-Keep-moving-inc-poster.ashx).

Good sleep hygiene should be advised. Dependent on their employment situation, methods for the patient to remain in work or to regain employment should be suggested.

Non-pharmacological options

Of the non-pharmacological treatments available, CBT appears to result in the most improvement for pain and function. There is now evidence to show that telephone CBT can also provide benefits, which is considered to be a cheaper option than face to face CBT. Online CBT may also be an option for some patients, or alternative 'talking therapies' as deemed appropriate according to the individual patient.

Encourage appropriate physical activity for the individual patient. If this is something that the patient currently struggles with then a graded exercise programme through physiotherapy referral could be considered. A recent study showed that the combination of an expert-led exercise programme and telephone CBT did not result in greater improvements than either option on its own.

Alternative therapies might be useful for some patients, although there is limited evidence to support these; suggestions include massage, acupuncture and balneotherapy.

Pharmacological options

These are only useful for some patients and should be tailored to specific symptoms. The evidence base suggests that the following are appropriate drugs to use; however, not all are licensed in the UK for pain relief.

Simple analgesics such as paracetamol and weak opioids (strong opioids and corticosteroids are not recommended). Tramadol has been shown to be effective to reduce fibromyalgia pain symptoms. NSAIDs have an effect on peripheral pain and as such are only useful for widespread pain patients if they have occurrences of peripheral pain, e.g. osteoarthritis alongside their widespread pain.

Antidepressants have been shown to reduce pain symptoms and improve function and have the benefit of improving depressive symptoms in patients with chronic pain. Amitryptiline has the most supporting evidence, while others, including fluoxetine, duloxetine, and moclobemide have also been found to be associated with improvements in pain. Drugs that help with sleep problems may also be useful, although these should be used for the shortest possible time and are not recommended for repeat medication. Anticonvulsant drugs gabapentin and pregabalin have been recommended, however there is limited evidence for these drugs and for their longer term benefit.

It is important to note that the majority of both the non-pharmacological and pharmacological therapies listed promote improvements in the short and medium term but there is less known about their long-term effects. Scheduling regular reviews to monitor the progress of a patient with widespread pain is recommended, with changes to management and further referral considered as appropriate.

Summary

Widespread musculoskeletal pain is complex and challenging for clinicians to manage. However, with a realistic and reassuring explanation alongside advice and support for the patient, symptoms can be managed. A combination of non-pharmacological and pharmacological treatments is recommended in order to successfully manage the patient in a holistic manner.

Further reading

Arthritis Research UK. *Clinical Assessment of the Musculoskeletal System – A Guide For Medical Students And Healthcare Professionals*. Arthritis Research UK, Chesterfield 2011. Available at: www.arthritisresearchuk.org/health -professionals-and-students/student-handbook.aspx (retrieved 30 July 2012).

Carville SF, Arendt-Nielsen S, Bliddal H, *et al*. EULAR evidence-based recommendations for the management of fibromyalgia syndrome. *Ann Rheum Dis* 2008;**67**(4):536–41.

Glennon P. *Fibromyalgia Syndrome: Management in Primary Care. Reports on the Rheumatic Diseases Series 6. Hands on No 7*. Arthritis Research UK, Chesterfield, 2010.

Map of Medicine. *Map of Medicine for Chronic Widespread Pain*. Available at: www.mapofmedicine.com (Accessed 26 April 2012).

McBeth J, Mulvey MR. Fibromyalgia: mechanisms, and potential impact of the ACR 2010 classification criteria. *Nat Rev Rheumatol* 2012;**8**(2):108–16.

Turk DC, Wilson HD. Managing fibromyalgia: an update on diagnosis and treatment. *J Musc Med* 2009;**10**:S1–7.

Wolfe F, Clauw DJ, Fitzcharles MA, *et al*. The American College of Rheumatology preliminary diagnostic criteria for fibromyalgia and measurement of symptom severity. *Arthritis Care Res (Hoboken)* 2010;**62**:600–10.

CHAPTER 12

Fatigue

Alison J. Wearden

School of Psychological Sciences, University of Manchester, Manchester, UK

> **OVERVIEW**
>
> - Some level of fatigue is very common in community surveys and in individuals who consult their GPs
> - Fatigue may be a consequence of a recognised physical illness, be the first indicator of a new illness or be a primary problem.
> - A diagnosis of chronic fatigue syndrome can be safely made in general practice following NICE guidelines

Epidemiology in primary care

Fatigue symptoms

Fatigue is a very common symptom associated with a wide range of medical conditions. Because fatigue is difficult to define and measure, estimates of the prevalence of fatigue tend to be imprecise. UK community surveys suggest that around 20% men and 30% women have suffered from 'always feeling tired' in the past month. Studies that have asked primary care attenders whether they have been troubled by fatigue find that 10 to 30% respond positively, although possibly as few as 1 in 10 of these will present with fatigue as their primary problem.

Many fatigued patients will have a medical condition that might account for their fatigue, but a quarter to a half will not. The prevalence of medically unexplained fatigue in UK primary care consulters has been variously estimated at around 10–15%. Epidemiological studies find that women are about 1.5 times more likely to be fatigued than men. The sex ratio is higher for cases with more severe or more chronic fatigue and lower if those with comorbid psychiatric disorders are excluded. Fatigue may be under-recognised in patients from Black and minority ethnic sections of the community.

Chronic fatigue syndrome

Chronic fatigue syndrome (CFS, also known as ME and usually abbreviated to CFS/ME), is a condition in which the principal complaint is severe, disabling fatigue unexplained by other medical conditions, of at least 6 months duration. CFS/ME is associated with high levels of impairment, and social and economic costs. Preliminary evidence suggests that both mood disturbance (depression and anxiety) and a tendency to a driven, 'all-or-nothing' approach to managing symptoms, are associated with the progression to a more chronic fatigue state. A number of sets of diagnostic criteria for CFS/ME have been developed, each providing difference prevalence estimates, but in the UK, the prevalence is usually quoted as 0.2–0.4% of the population. Thus, many more patients experience unexplained sustained fatigue than meet the requirements for a diagnosis of CFS/ME.

GP assessment

Fatigue is a subjective feeling like pain, and is not directly measurable. Unlike some symptoms in this book, fatigue is a feeling familiar to us all. Studies in the general population have shown that fatigue lies on a continuum. Fatigue becomes a problem when it is experienced out of proportion to the level of exertion or work undertaken, and when it reaches a certain level of severity, chronicity and impact on a person's life. It is perhaps because fatigue is so familiar that it is not always recognised and treated.

GPs should take complaints of persistent fatigue seriously, not only because fatigue may be a symptom of a condition that requires treatment, but also because it is so distressing, and can become chronic and very disabling.

The term medically unexplained is somewhat misleading because it suggests that fatigue in the context of other conditions is medically explained. In fact, even when fatigue is an established feature of a condition, the causes and processes underlying fatigue are often poorly understood – to this extent, all fatigue is unexplained. Furthermore, programmes for treating fatigue in conditions such as cancer, rheumatoid arthritis, multiple sclerosis, and post-stroke tend to adopt the same approaches as those that are successful in managing medically unexplained fatigue, suggesting that the explained/unexplained distinction is not always very illuminating.

Typical features of functional symptoms

In primary care samples, severity of fatigue is strongly associated with distress. In the case of CFS/ME, fatigue is usually accompanied by muscle pain, sleep disturbance (hypersomnia, insomnia,

ABC of Medically Unexplained Symptoms, First Edition.
Edited by Christopher Burton.

disturbed sleep–wake cycles, and waking unrefreshed), mood disturbance, and memory and concentration problems (often termed 'mental fatigue'). Other symptoms and syndromes are also commonly associated with fatigue, such as dizziness, nausea and malaise, and the symptoms of IBS.

Certain infections, for example glandular fever, place patients at greater risk of developing prolonged fatigue, but a substantial minority of patients with prolonged fatigue are unable to pinpoint any particular trigger. Patients with sleep problems often report daytime fatigue, but in some cases may actually be experiencing excessive daytime sleepiness. It is important to consider whether fatigue is secondary to poor sleep (including poor sleep due to depression). In many cases, however, fatigue coexists with normal or increased sleep, although that sleep may be experienced as unrefreshing.

Typical features of organic symptoms and red flag symptoms

Fatigue is non-specific, and is known to be associated with many medical conditions. In fact, patients with fatiguing conditions (such as rheumatoid arthritis, multiple sclerosis and even cancer) often say that fatigue is their most troubling symptom. In terms of what it feels like for the patient, there is no easy way to distinguish fatigue that is a symptom of one of these conditions from fatigue that is not – that is, fatigue may feel similar whatever is underlying it.

In order to rule out other possible causes of fatigue, look for additional signs and symptoms that may be associated with those other conditions. The NICE guidelines for CFS/ME identify a number of 'red flag' features that should always be investigated. These are listed in Box 12.1.

Box 12.1 Red flag features indicating possible serious causes for fatigue

- Localising/focal neurological signs
- Signs and symptoms of inflammatory arthritis or connective tissue disease
- Signs and symptoms of cardiorespiratory disease
- Significant weight loss
- Sleep apnoea
- Clinically significant lymphadenopathy

History and examination tips

Take a careful history including when the fatigue started, and the context in which it now occurs, including social and occupational stressors. Ask about sleep, and consider whether you need to rule out sleep apnoea (particularly if patients fall asleep inappropriately). Enquire about any prescription or non-prescription drugs that the patient may be taking, as these may cause fatigue. Some patients who have been fatigued for many years may have a complicated history, and may need to be assessed over more than one appointment.

Listen to the patient and try to understand the way in which they view their fatigue. A significant minority of patients will have comorbid depression and/or anxiety disorders, which should be treated as sympathetically as if they would be if they were the primary problem.

Referral and investigations

The NICE guidelines for CFS/ME also provide a number of diagnostic tests that should normally be carried out by the GP (see Box 12.2), as well as a list of tests that are not usually advised – these include serological testing.

Box 12.2 Tests that should usually be carried out in order to exclude other conditions

- Urinalysis for protein, blood and glucose
- Full blood count
- Urea and electrolytes
- Liver function
- Thyroid function
- Erythrocyte sedimentation rate or plasma viscosity
- C-reactive protein
- Random blood glucose
- Serum creatinine
- Screening blood tests for gluten sensitivity
- Serum calcium
- Creatine kinase

Scenario 1

'Jane' is a 38-year-old Macmillan Nurse and mother who feels tired all the time and thinks this may have started after an episode of gastroenteritis several months ago. She is finding it hard, because of the fatigue, to cope with her multiple roles. She has no red flag symptoms or signs but seems almost tearful during interview. Her GP thinks she is probably physically and emotionally exhausted but carries out routine investigations.

Blood tests reveal marked hypothyroidism.

Clinical decision

The NICE guidelines for CFS/ME recommend that, if the patient has been fatigued for 4 months (3 months in children and young people) and other diagnoses have been ruled out, a diagnosis of CFS/ME can be made. The diagnosis should be reconsidered if none of the following features are present: post-exertional fatigue or malaise, cognitive difficulties, sleep disturbance, pain.

Explanation

Having had other potential causes of fatigue ruled out by tests, patients with medically unexplained fatigue are often left feeling that no explanation is being offered for their troubling symptoms; this can lead them to feel disbelieved, fearful that there is an underlying disease that has been missed, and, distressingly, that there is nothing that can be done to help them. It is therefore very important to tell patients that in fact we do have an explanation for their symptoms, and then to confidently provide that explanation in terms that are acceptable to patients.

In patients with mild or relatively recent (less than 3 months) fatigue it is reasonable to take an optimistic line as most individuals recover fully.

Feeling exhausted like this is sometimes nature's way of saying you need to catch up with yourself. Everyone's body has ways of making them feel like this and because it is a natural process the tests for disease are all OK. As this is a relatively recent thing, then concentrate on getting plenty of sleep and looking after yourself. Try to make some time to do things you enjoy, including gentle exercise; it's likely that you will find the energy coming back.

In more severe and persistent fatigue, it is often useful to start by suggesting that the factors that precipitated the fatigue (for example, another illness, overwork, response to psychological stressors, or unidentifiable factors), are unlikely to be the same as those that are perpetuating it.

You've told me that your fatigue started after you had flu last winter. At the time, you were under a lot of pressure at work, as well as having to look after your mother when she broke her hip, and you probably didn't have the time to rest and recover properly. You were still feeling so tired and ill 8 weeks after you started with the flu that you would come home from work and go straight to bed. Gradually, you found yourself doing less and less outside of the essentials – work and looking after other people. You started to lose fitness, your muscles started to weaken, and, not surprisingly, you became quite demoralised. All this happened over a period of time, long after the bout of flu had ended, but you were feeling worse and worse.

Patients are often unaware that too much rest can be counterproductive, both in terms of cardiovascular and muscular deconditioning and other effects. Furthermore, once patients have become relatively deconditioned, an increase in activity is likely to lead to unpleasant symptoms, such as muscle soreness (which may be delayed for 48–72 h). If an increase in symptoms is interpreted as a sign of damage or relapse, and the patient responds by taking more rest, a vicious cycle, or downward spiral is set up.

Another common pattern is for patients with a rather all-or-nothing approach to life to attempt to do too much on 'good days', only to crash and need to spend several days resting; this vacillating pattern can obscure a general downward trend.

There is quite good evidence that when fit and healthy people are forced to be inactive, particularly if they are confined to bed, they soon become deconditioned; they are less able to deliver oxygen to their muscles to power activity, they may suffer from dizziness when they stand up, temperature regulation can be affected, and it becomes harder to concentrate. Also, if people who have been resting attempt to get back to previous levels of activity too quickly, due to muscular deconditioning, they can experience quite severe muscle soreness, which can come on 2–3 days after the activity. The best way to avoid all this is to do a little activity every day and to build up activity levels very gradually.

Two other features of fatigue that can be explained to patients, if relevant, are disturbed sleep–wake cycles and the (potentially reversible) dysregulation of the hypothalamo–pituitary–adrenal (HPA) axis.

Paradoxically, being inactive can make you feel more tired and sleepy. If you find yourself falling asleep during the day, it is unlikely that you will sleep as well at night. Then you may wake up after a few hours, or wake up in the morning feeling unrefreshed. Related to this, poor sleep and lower levels of activity are associated with disturbance in what is called the HPA axis – a system that prepares the body to be active. We know that some chronically fatigued patients have low levels of circulating cortisol that might contribute to their tiredness, but it appears that this state of affairs can be reversed by a gradual return to more normal activity levels.

Finally it is important to explain that if a patient is relatively deconditioned, she or he can expect a slight increase in symptoms as activity levels are increased, but that these symptoms are normal and to be expected, and not a sign of damage to the body or relapse.

Scenario 2

'Angela' is a 39-year-old office manager, currently working reduced hours because of her illness, who presented with over 6 months of disabling fatigue. Her GP carried out the investigations shown in Box 12.2, which were normal, and felt confident in making a diagnosis of chronic fatigue syndrome. Angela agreed to referral for CBT.

The initial sessions focused on agreeing the nature of Angela's problem and identifying her short-, medium- and long-term goals for recovery. She and her therapist then agreed a phased programme of re-introducing activities that Angela had dropped. Although Angela was initially fearful of provoking a relapse of her symptoms, with the help of her therapist, she learned that fluctuations in fatigue and muscle pain were a normal part of her recovery. After eight sessions of CBT, Angela was able to increase her working hours to 80% and was also enjoying leisure activities with her family.

Specific treatment

A good evidence base for treating CFS/ME has started to accumulate, and it is now clear that the two treatments that have proven efficacy for the management of CFS/ME are CBT and graded-exercise therapy (GET), when carried out by experienced therapists with a good knowledge and understanding of CFS/ME. What is *not* helpful in terms of recovery, is limiting activities to conserve energy – this limits symptoms in the short term, but will contribute to declining levels of functional ability in the long term. Although there is less evidence about the treatment of sub-syndromal unexplained fatigue states, what there is suggests that severe and less chronic fatigue symptoms will respond to similar management approaches as does CFS/ME. The NICE guidelines recommend that management based on the principles of CBT and GET is started early.

The key factors in management of unexplained fatigue are to engage the patient by believing them and instilling confidence in them, to provide an explanation for symptoms in terms of the vicious cycle outlined above, and then to collaboratively work out a programme of very gradually increasing activity. It is very important not to simply suggest that the patient does more exercise – this advice is likely to lead to a relapse of symptoms and the reinforcement of the idea that activity is harmful to the body. Instead, a gradual, controlled programme should be devised, starting at a level that the patient can currently easily manage. Other advice might relate to good sleep management and scheduling periods of rest. Dietary advice should emphasise a normal well-balanced diet with regular meals. There is some evidence that the needs of carers of patients with more severe fatigue are not being addressed.

There is no recommended pharmacological treatment for unexplained fatigue. Antidepressants and analgesics are often prescribed for symptom relief but should be used with caution and reviewed regularly. For patients with CFS/ME, the possibility of referral for specialist care should be discussed within 6 months of presentation, if there is no improvement in symptoms. As noted earlier, CBT delivered by a cognitive behavioural therapist or GET, often delivered by a physiotherapist or occupational therapist, are the treatments with the best evidence base. Both treatments should be discussed with patients and the referral made on the basis of a consideration of the patients symptoms, physical and cognitive functioning and preference.

Conclusion

Mild and transient forms of fatigue are relatively common in primary care and should be taken seriously with appropriate examination, investigation and explanation. If tests are negative it is important to take an optimistic line, to encourage a sensible balance of rest and activity, and to reassure that most cases resolve spontaneously. Some patients with severe and persistent fatigue meet recognised criteria for CFS/ME and are more likely to respond to CBT or GET than to usual care or other currently tested interventions.

For additional advice on the management of relapse and setbacks, and on helping patients with severe CFS/ME, see the NICE guidelines.

Further reading

Burgess M, Chalder T. *Overcoming Chronic Fatigue*. Robinson Publishing, London, 2005.

National Institute for Health and Clinical Excellence. *Chronic Fatigue Syndrome/Myalgic Encephalomyelitis (or Encephalopathy): Diagnosis and Management. Clinical Guideline CG53*. NICE, London, 2007.

Pemberton S, Berry C. *Fighting Fatigue. Overcoming the Symptoms of CFS/ME*. Hammersmith Press, London, 2009.

Wessely S, Hotopf M, Sharpe, M. *Chronic Fatigue and its Syndromes*. Oxford University Press, Oxford, 1988.

CHAPTER 13

Neurological Symptoms: Weakness, Blackouts and Dizziness

Jon Stone[1] and Alan Carson[2]

[1]Department of Clinical Neurosciences, Western General Hospital, Edinburgh, UK
[1]Robert Fergusson Unit, University of Edinburgh, Edinburgh, UK

OVERVIEW

- The assessment of whether weakness and blackouts are due to a neurological disease process is not easy and usually requires referral to a neurologist. Dizziness is easier to assess in primary care
- The diagnosis of most functional neurological symptoms should be made on the basis of positive evidence in the examination, for example incongruity and inconsistency of limb weakness, not on the absence of disease and normal investigations
- Dizziness can be usefully divided into light-headedness, vertigo and dissociation
- A transparent and effective initial approach to diagnosis, explanation and treatment is possible

---

Introduction

Around one in six patients referred from primary care to neurology have physical symptoms that turn out not to be due to a disease, which we shall refer to as functional symptoms in this chapter. An additional one in six patients have a mixture of neurological disease and functional symptoms.

Functional neurological symptoms, also known as conversion disorder, psychogenic/non-organic/dissociative neurological symptoms, present a particular challenge in primary care because specialist knowledge and investigations are often required to make the diagnosis. However, the bulk of patient management takes place in primary care and, unfortunately many patients are returned from secondary care without adequate follow-up or treatment. So awareness of how the diagnosis should be made and modes of treatment therefore remain important for all doctors.

Functional weakness

Epidemiology

Functional weakness is one of the commonest causes of limb weakness in patients under the age of 50, with a mean age of

onset of 39. It is at least as common as multiple sclerosis. Patients with this diagnosis will, according to studies, turn out to have a disease explanation at follow-up in less than 5% of cases, a frequency that parallels all other neurological and psychiatric disorders.

Clinical features of functional weakness

Patients with functional weakness most commonly complain of weakness of one side of their body, often with a feeling that the limb does not feel part of them; they drop things or their knee keeps giving way. Typically they have a history of other functional symptoms, especially pain, fatigue and concentration problems. In 50% they have a sudden 'stroke-like' onset, often with panic, symptoms of dissociation (see below) or a physical injury. The diagnosis should not be based on the presence or absence of stressful life events, which are less common than the name 'conversion disorder' suggests.

Scenario 1

'Martin' is a 41-year-old information technology worker who had been admitted on several occasions to hospital for left-sided weakness. He was discharged with a normal MRI head scan and no diagnosis but continues to feel that something is wrong in his left arm and leg. He also feels unusually tired and can't concentrate. He wonders if he has been having mini-strokes and is starting to think that doctors don't believe him. He has a history of anxiety in the past but says that recently he has not been under stress at all.

The diagnosis can be suspected from the history but should only be made on the basis of the physical examination. In this respect functional weakness differs somewhat from symptoms such as pain and fatigue where the examination is much less helpful.

The key finding is of inconsistency of movement, for example a patient who cannot move their ankles on the bed but who can stand on tiptoes and heels. A useful, more repeatable test for patients with leg weakness is Hoover's sign (Figure 13.1). Although developed as a test to 'trick' patients, it can be usefully shared with patients to show them how they have a problem with voluntary movement that improves with distraction (and therefore must be due to a problem in nervous system functioning rather than damage). A dragging gait is also quite specific for more severe functional

---

ABC of Medically Unexplained Symptoms, First Edition.
Edited by Christopher Burton.

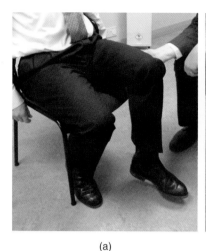
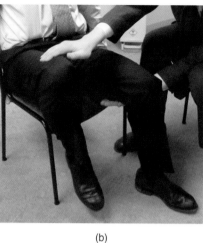

(a)   (b)

Figure 13.1 Hoovers sign – a clinical sign of functional weakness. (a) Test hip extension – it is weak. (b) Test contralateral hip flexion against resistance – hip extension has become strong.

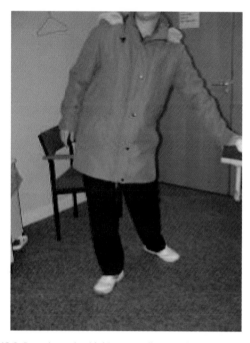

Figure 13.2 Dragging gait with hip externally rotated typical of functional weakness.

paralysis (Figure 13.2). Other less reliable pointers to functional weakness include a global pattern of weakness in the limb, sensory disturbance that stops at the shoulder or groin and 'give way' weakness in which the limb 'gives way' to light pressure but can return to normal with encouragement.

GP assessment

Limb weakness may, of course, have many causes. The commonest in the age group typically affected are multiple sclerosis and stroke but a large number of rarer conditions need to be considered, which is why referral to a neurologist is usually advisable. Weakness may accompany migraine but should resolve within 24 h.

Referral is usually indicated for functional weakness for several reasons. These are relatively uncommon problems and need skilled assessment. Furthermore some patients may have both functional weakness and a structural 'organic' neurological disease and investigation may still be needed.

In referring a patient it may be reasonable to suggest (to patient and specialist) that you suspect a functional disorder and include information about the patient's psychological state. However, it is wrong to assume either that weakness is functional because of the presence of a psychiatric diagnosis or that it cannot be functional because the patient is psychologically 'normal'.

Explanation

A helpful explanation for functional weakness includes giving the patient a diagnosis that emphasises that the symptoms are relatively common, genuine and potentially reversible. Explanation alone sometimes leads to recovery. Wherever possible explain to the patient the way in which the diagnosis has been made. The use of metaphor and self-help material (e.g.www.neurosymptoms.org) is often helpful.

You have functional weakness, a common and potentially reversible problem. Your leg is weak when you are trying to move it but the power actually comes back to normal when you are distracted by moving your good leg. This is called Hoover's Sign. The sign shows that your brain is having trouble sending a message to move to the leg, but the fact it can temporarily return to normal shows it is not damaged. It's like a software problem on a computer rather than a hardware problem. Its important for you to know that, even though I know this is all a bit strange, I believe you and I don't think you're imagining the problem.

Specific treatment

Further treatment may involve psychologically informed physiotherapy/graded exercise for patients with disabling weakness. In the absence of these, encouraging patients to work through a self-help approach and using the principles outlined in this book can be effective.

Blackouts/dissociative (non-epileptic attacks)

Epidemiology

Around one in seven patients attending a 'first fit' clinic and up to 50% of patients brought into hospital have a diagnosis of non-epileptic attacks, also called pseudoseizures, psychogenic non-epileptic attacks and dissociative non-epileptic attacks.

Clinical features of dissociative (non-epileptic) attacks

Attacks commonly consist either of generalised shaking, an episode in which the patient suddenly falls down and lies still or a 'blank spell'.

Patients often do not spontaneously report warning symptoms and rarely report episodes triggered by specific stressful events. With closer questioning, symptoms of panic and dissociation can commonly be found that the patient is reluctant to divulge, partly because they do not want to think about it and partly because they do not want to be considered 'crazy'.

Scenario 2

'Helen' is a 23-year-old shop assistant who keeps having attacks at random at work. She said they rarely happen at home. She initially couldn't recall any warning symptoms but with some prompting admitted she tended to feel scared and dizzy just before them, just long enough to go to a store room where she blacks out and shakes for 2–3 min. Work colleagues describe how she shakes violently for several minutes before coming round.

Table 13.1 gives some clinical clues to the diagnosis of attack disorders. Witness histories tend to be inaccurate and can be misleading. Many specialists will aim to obtain a video electroencephalogram (EEG) capturing a usual attack, which is the gold standard investigation.

GP assessment

As for functional weakness the principles of referral and sharing your diagnostic thoughts should be based on what happens during the attack rather than psychological factors.

Explanation

A helpful explanation for dissociative non-epileptic attacks includes giving the patient a diagnosis that emphasises that the symptoms are common, genuine and potentially reversible. There is excellent self-help information available (e.g. www.nonepilepticattacks.info).

> *You have dissociative non-epileptic attacks, a common and potentially reversible problem. We know from the video they recorded at the hospital that your attacks are typical for this diagnosis and also that there was no evidence of abnormal electrical activity on the EEG that you would see in epilepsy. Dissociative attacks (which are also called non-epileptic attacks) are a trance-like state, a bit like being suddenly hypnotised. They usually occur out of the blue although some patients can experience frightening symptoms of feeling 'spaced out' or 'not with it' just before they black out – these feelings are called dissociation. It's important for you to know that, even though I know this is all a bit strange, I believe you and I don't think you're imaging the problem.*

CBT using distraction techniques appears to be effective for non-epileptic attacks. There is no clear evidence regarding antidepressants.

Dizziness

Epidemiology in primary care

Dizziness is a common presenting symptom in primary care that often induces hopelessness in the clinician. The reported prevalence

---

Table 13.1 Clinical features that help (or do not help) to differentiate dissociative (non-epileptic) attacks from generalized tonic-clonic epileptic seizures and syncope.

	Dissociative attacks	Epileptic seizures	Syncope
Helpful features			
Fall down and lie still for >30 s	Common	Very rare	Very rare
Duration >2 min	Common	Rare	Very rare
Eyes and mouth closed	Common	Rare	Rare
Resisting eye opening	Common	Very rare	Very rare
Side-to-side head or body movement	Common	Rare	Rare
Visible large bite mark on side of tongue/cheek/lip	Very rare	Occasional	Rare
Grunting/Guttural 'ictal cry' sound	Rare	Common	Rare
Weeping/upset after a seizure	Occasional	Very rare	Rare
Recall for period of unresponsiveness	Common	Very rare	Very rare
Thrashing, violent movements	Common	Rare	Rare
Attacks in medical situations	Common	Rare	Rare
Unhelpful features			
Attack arising from sleep	Occasional	Common	Rare
Aura	Common	Common	Common
Incontinence of urine	Occasional	Common	Common
Injury	Common	Common	Common
Report of tongue biting	Common	Common	Common

Table 13.2 What do patients mean by the word 'dizzy'? – types of dizziness and common causes.

Symptom	'Does it feel like . . . ?'	Common causes
Vertigo	'. . . a sensation of movement even though you are still? Is it made worse with movement?'	Benign paroxysmal positional vertigo (BPPV) Migrainous vertigo Labyrinthitis Ménière's disease Minor head trauma
Light-headedness	'. . . a faint feeling as if you might pass out? Do you feel hot with it?'	Orthostatic/cardiac/vasovagal hypotensionHyperventilation
Dysequilibrium	'. . . a feeling that your whole body is unsteady that is worse if you are standing or walking?'	'Chronic subjective dizziness' Phobic postural vertigo
Dissociation	. . . as if you are 'spaced out', 'there but not there' or 'disconnected' from things?'	Anxiety Fatigue states

of dizziness in the community is huge with around 20% of adults and 30% or more of older adults reporting the symptom.

GP assessment

Try to find out what the patient means by dizziness using one or more of the four categories in Table 13.2. The nature of the dizziness will help narrow down the cause of the problem, although often there will be more than one (Table 13.2). Physical assessment, e.g. the Dix–Hallpike test, stepping test, lying, standing blood pressure will depend on the nature of the symptom.

> ### Scenario 3
>
> 'Lindsey' is a 19-year-old girl who 2 years after an illness labelled as 'labyrinthitis' with vertigo has developed incapacitating dizziness. She finds it hard to describe but it is a mixture of general unsteadiness and wobbliness mixed with scary dissociative symptoms of feeling spaced out. It is not true vertigo because it is not really worse with moving or a sensation of movement when still. She feels particularly dizzy when she is outside or when looking at patterned surfaces. As a consequence she has become frightened to leave the house and worried about a sinister cause.

Typical features of functional dizziness

Vestibular problems are common. As in the case scenario, patients with functional dizziness often have a history of a conventional cause of vertigo such as migraine, benign paroxysmal positional vertigo (BPPV) or an episode of acute vestibulopathy (often called labyrinthitis without good evidence).

Altered signals from the 'ill' vestibular system clash with signals from the other, healthy, vestibular system creating vertigo. Normally the brain will gradually adapt to the change and vertigo will disappear. However, in patients with chronic subjective dizziness the whole experience leaves them with an overawareness of their own balance systems, which the patient tends to anxiously monitor for a recurrence and then the problem persists.

Anxiety, agoraphobia, hyperventilation, fatigue and dissociative symptoms can easily follow (see Figure 13.3). 'Chronic subjective dizziness', 'phobic postural vertigo' and 'space and motion discomfort' all refer to symptoms in this complex. Neck pain is

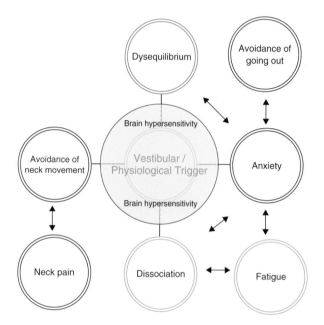

Figure 13.3 How a minor self-limiting vestibular disturbance can result in chronic dizziness and anxiety.

also common in patients with persistent dizziness because head movements tend to be avoided.

Explanation

Explanation in this situation is about unpicking the various factors in Figure 13.3 in a way that the patient can start to see how they might start to 'turn the volume knob down' on their dizzy sensations. This can be achieved by recognising that symptoms such as dissociation are intensified both by attention paid to them and by anxiety about dizziness.

Treatment

Vestibular exercises may be helpful even in patients without true vertigo. CBT for anxiety, ideally with a therapist who understands the links to dizziness, may also help. Patients will tend to be very sensitive to side effects of medication.

Further reading

Hallett M, Cloninger CR, Fahn S, *et al. Psychogenic Movement Disorders and Other Conversion Disorders.* Cambridge University Press, Cambridge, 2011.

Schacter S, LaFrance WC. (2010). *Gates and Rowan's Nonepileptic Seizures.* Cambridge University Press, Cambridge, 2010.

Stone J. The bare essentials – functional symptoms in neurology. *Pract Neurol* 2009;**9**:179 – 89.

Williams C, Carson A, Kent C, *et al. Overcoming Functional Neurological Symptoms.* Hodder, London, 2011.

www.neurosymptoms.org – a self-help website for patients with functional and dissociative neurological symptoms.

www.nonepilepticattacks.info – a self-help website for patients with non-epileptic attacks.

CHAPTER 14

Managing Medically Unexplained Symptoms in The Consultation

Avril F. Danczak

Central and South Manchester Speciality Training Programme for General Practice, North Western Deanery and The Alexandra Practice, Manchester, UK

> **OVERVIEW**
>
> - Enhanced consultation skills enable doctors to work with patients with medically unexplained symptoms (MUS) in creative, personalised and effective ways
> - Deep listening and empathy strengthen the therapeutic value of the doctor – patient relationship
> - Effective consultations lead to constructive explanations and translate them into therapeutic alliance and actions

Introduction

'*Thanks for listening*'. Doctors are delighted when patients use this phrase, describing an apparently simple process. Such thanks can be a sign of the most powerful and satisfying processes in medicine. If patients feel understood and accepted, then healing, changes in behaviour and effective management of their illness are all more probable. Yet listening deeply and effectively turns out to be neither simple nor easy to achieve. Indeed, listening itself is easy to understand, but hard to explain.

In this chapter, the skills needed to listen to patients with MUS will be explored; including getting the consultation started on the right footing, how to use 'deep' listening skills to enhance mutual understanding and acceptance, and how to develop personalised strategies for managing symptoms. Finally, additional techniques, useful for all patients are described.

All doctors set out to listen. So why is it sometimes so hard? And why does it sometimes go wrong? Here is a typical case history.

> **Scenario 1**
>
> '*Sarah*' *is a 39-year-old woman attending for follow-up 6 weeks after a seemingly routine laparoscopic cholecystectomy. She asks for a sick note as she can't face work because of pain: a 'burning indigestion feeling in the tummy', she feels fatigued and exhausted, nauseated*

> *and unable to attend to normal activities, or even do yoga, which she usually enjoys. 'Why doesn't anyone do anything?'*
>
> *The doctor explores the pain in detail, asks about worries and concerns 'I just want to get back to normal' and offers analgesics. ' I have tried them at home and they are useless'. A thorough examination is normal, with a well healed scar.*
>
> *'Then why do I still feel so terrible? Can't you get rid of the pain?' Finally, the doctor offers a trial of a PPI (thinking it may be heartburn), a midstream urine sample to rule out infection, and an early follow-up appointment. After 20 min (it seemed shorter), Sarah leaves the room saying 'You just haven't listened to me at all'.*

The doctor has tried hard, given lots of time and slumps back exhausted wondering what else she could do.

Similar scenarios will have been encountered by most doctors. Sometimes things just do not work out in one consultation. By arranging an early follow-up, this doctor has shown a key commitment to their continuing relationship.

Getting the consultation off to a good start

Doctors can be ambivalent about patients with MUS. Patients may also feel uneasy, picking up that they are not welcome or fearing dismissive approaches. This leads to mutual frustration. Anticipate a positive experience, and prepare yourself to attend to what the patient is saying in an open and relaxed way. Greet patients warmly and by name, show you remember them (e.g. by remembering a telling detail, or an event they have mentioned). If it is a follow-up, thank them for coming back to see you.

Think about your opening statement. Asking 'how can I help' may be doomed to failure as you often cannot do what the patient wishes for. When people come with new problems, your silence will leave a gap for their opening statements. With MUS, especially at follow-up, it may be more helpful to focus on the patient's perceptions of priority. Thus, 'What would you like to prioritise/talk about /focus on/today?'.

Explore the pros and cons of different openings in your own consultations. Try different approaches at different times and see what works best; most patients with MUS will be seeing you a few times. Adding your own agenda items ('I would also like to check on the progress of your diabetes') means that you create space to treat the treatable and ensure that chronic disease is attended to fully. This is important when MUS coexists with medical conditions.

If you are picking up from a previous consultation, specifically ask about progress with the agreed management plan. Listen carefully for the emotional and cognitive content. Use opportunities to show empathy and kindness whenever possible. The practical strategies in Box 14.1 can demonstrate your commitment to, and interest in the patient's distress.

Box 14.1 **Enhancing listening skills at the start of the consultation**

- Have a repertoire of opening statements. Observe what works best for you
- Develop your listening skills by videoing a consultation with the patient's permission. Watch it alone or with a colleague, stopping every minute to describe and digest WHAT the patient is saying, HOW they are saying it, what they are NOT saying
- Note down sentences that the patient used and then discuss them with a colleague. The better you listen the more is remembered
- Thinking in detail about cues improves doctors' understanding. This can turn a 'snapshot' of a patient into a 'chapter from a novel'. For instance 'I am OK when I start the day, but after 2 hours at work with the door banging and all those people I am just exhausted again'. Find out what is going on in those 2 hours, and what drags the patient down
- Share your thoughts about the patient with them. Sometimes this 'meta communication' or 'thinking about thinking' can help unstick a situation

---

Deep listening skills

The skills of 'deep listening' (also called 'enhanced listening') help doctors to achieve a closer understanding of the patients' illness and of their suffering. Many patients with MUS feel that they are not treated respectfully or taken seriously. All too often they feel dismissed or unheard. Listening deeply means attending to, and remembering everything the patient communicates. Use encouraging skills ('go on', 'tell me more', or' please tell me the details') rather than a barrage of questions. Clarifying details after the patient has finished speaking (avoiding interruptions) will demonstrate your interest. Show that you accept what they are experiencing via empathic comments ('So the burning night pain really affects your sleep').

Try emphasising the 'feel' in the question, 'what does it feel like?'. Then listen carefully to what the patient chooses to communicate with you. Sometimes an evocative description will follow ('it is really like a knife going in '), sometimes a concern (' it feels like it is going to burst'), or maybe an insight into their despair and fear ('It feels as if it will never give me any peace!').

When summarising or reflecting back, reflect the overt content ('so the back pain never leaves you, and it's a severe jabbing sort of pain') and the emotional overtones ('you are concerned it will never get any better, so you won't enjoy your grandchildren').

Less is more

Rather than asking many medically focused questions, reflect back the words the patient uses. This usually stimulates more detail.

Patient: *I told the consultant that it still hurts after the surgery, but he just fobbed me off.*

Doctor: *Fobbed you off?*

Patient: *Yes . . . that well . . . it made me . . . made me wonder . . . perhaps something went wrong inside.*

Doctor: *Went wrong inside?*

Patient: *Yes, with the op, maybe he left something there.*

These specific ideas can then be used when creating explanations, and using the patient's own exact words later on will increase engagement. Explanations are more credible if they pick up on the patient's own words and ideas. In the above situation, explanations could reflect the fact that restoration and repair processes can be uncomfortable or distressing too. Highlighting emotive terms ('it feels like you are all blocked up?') or terms that indicate the impact on them ('So you can't go out because you will need to go to the loo all the time') will also help the patient to feel understood and accepted.

Using non-verbal (body language) and paraverbal (tone of voice) information

Be aware of minimal clues to the patient's thoughts and feelings. For example, minor hesitations, looking away, the tone and loudness of their speech, may all speak volumes about their state of mind. Empathising with the feelings they express ('you seem a bit hesitant . . .') validates their experiences. Can their underlying anger, frustration or disappointment be verbalised? Patients often express a need for an explanation. This can be put to good use, as the doctor can lead into one of the explanatory models described in other chapters.

Exploit the paraverbal aspects of your own communications to patients; a kindly tone of voice, attentive body language, making the patient comfortable during examinations etc.

Picking up when listening is not working

At times the sensitive doctor will be aware of signs that rapport is being lost; changing approaches will help to avoid frustrating repetition and conflict where the doctor and patient have different views and goals.

Box 14.2 **Signs that listening is going wrong**

- Patients repeating the same information over and over again; this means they do not yet feel they are being heard (Repetition)
- The addition of new symptoms alongside the ones you are already considering (Expansion)
- Symptom descriptions seeming to get more florid (Amplification)

When this happens try a different approach. Consider that there may be an unspoken message, an unarticulated anxiety, symptoms that have underlying serious meaning to the patient, but which you have not yet appreciated. Empathic statements, rather than further questions, can show patients that they are accompanied and subtly change the direction.

Mirroring the patients posture can help you to appreciate what they are feeling, and also help them to know you are 'with them' emotionally.

Scenario 1 *(continued)*

Sarah did come back. Stung by the accusation of 'not listening' the doctor resolved to 'simply listen', signalling this to the patient by letting Sarah talk without interruption, avoiding questions, and simply repeating a few of her key words in any pauses.

Sarah: *I don't feel well enough to go back to work, but I need to get on.*
Doctor: *Get on?*
Sarah: *Yes, it's only me that has any ambition.*
Doctor: *Ambition?*

Sarah then poured out her frustrations; the responsibility for the family seemed to rest on her, her husband wouldn't go for promotion, was too timid, she had to be the one to increase the family income, after her operation she couldn't summon up the energy, she feared her own job would be at risk if she stayed off too long, but the pain was still bad.

After 10 min (it felt much longer) she stood up and said 'thank you for listening' and went back to work 3 days later.

Avoiding the problem of 'The doctor thinks I am imagining it'

Remember that although there may be common causes between MUS and vulnerability to emotional disorder, MUS frequently occur without a clear cut underlying emotional upset. It is important to avoid simplistic links to distress and encompass the full variety of symptoms. Understanding the patient's experience enables the doctor to choose an explanatory model that picks up on the words and concepts the patient uses themselves. Such explanations are neutral in content, do not imply that the patient is 'at fault' (emotionally or behaviourally) and can lead to joint decisions about helpful interventions. ('As your bowel is quite tight and tense, the medicine that relaxes the rhythm and makes it more regular will ease the spasms'). See the symptom chapters for fuller details about good explanatory models to use.

Examination with commentary

When examining, explain as you go along and use positive language where appropriate. Offer 'a full (or proper) examination', rather than 'a quick look', which may sound careless to the patient. Explain what/how you are 'thoroughly checking' (e.g. heart rate, rhythm, sounds, checking for murmurs.) Use ideas that the patient has mentioned and show that you have them in mind. 'I am checking for a blockage now' or 'You mentioned a tear, but you are showing me the muscle working well and strongly, so it is not torn'.

Use words like 'normal, healthy, strong' where appropriate. These words are better than saying 'there's nothing abnormal here' or 'I can't particularly find anything wrong' that could sound dismissive to the patient. Such phrases may even imply that you are not competent to find out what is wrong, and patients may interpret this to mean there is something hidden or even sinister happening to them.

It can be useful to explain 'technical' phenomena such as allodynia or hyperalgesia, where a light, non-damaging touch is interpreted by oversensitive nerve fibres as pain. This takes practice to get right, but is worthwhile because it shows that you are making sense of the patient's account, and recognising the reality of their experiences. Demonstrate and explain how you are testing for allodynia or hyperalgesia: for example a light skin pinch over the abdominal wall may reproduce the pain.

So, it felt very sore when I pressed on your abdomen, and then when I squeezed the skin there you still felt the pain. That tells me that the all the pain nerves in this area are turned up too high and are very sensitive.

Breaking good news

An effective examination for a presumed functional disorder will include explanation and feedback as you go along. For some patients this will be enough to reassure them. However, investigations may still be needed to rule out conditions of concern to the doctor, and at times, to exclude something the patient has expressed a specific concern about. The symptom chapters in this book suggest when this is the case and include guidelines on what to test. If you are carrying out tests to rule out unlikely conditions then say so. Explain in advance if you are anticipating normal tests.

We need to rule out a couple of conditions here [with appropriate explanation, and referring to any conditions the patient has concerns about]. If the tests are normal as we anticipate, we will both be reassured. Then we can concentrate on what we need to do to help you.

When you have concluded that the problem is (or is very likely to be) functional, breaking good news can still be a challenge. Saying that the tests are normal (or 'negative') is not enough and may leave patients even more puzzled about what could be wrong. This sometimes leads to a desire for more tests and an unhelpful spiral of investigation and failure of reassurance. Let patients have their results with a positive explanation.

Good, the bloods are normal, which tells me that what we thought is right, this should settle with time. The medication and exercise will help the healing process.

Explanations have been described in more detail in both the Principles of Assessment and Treatment (Chapter 6) and the specific symptom chapters. Remember that using patients exact words and concerns during explanations works better than jargon. Use explanations that accept distress, and also encourage expectations of healing and improvement. ('Wear and repair', 'spasm and relaxation', 'tightness and loosening' are useful phrases).

Always allow pauses for information to be digested. Pause after asking what questions the patient has. Check their responses to any suggestions, modifying your plans in the light of their understanding or ideas. Although no single approach will 'cure' all MUS, the skills outlined here will improve patient and doctor satisfaction.

Planning care and follow-up

Appropriate explanation can lead to creative interventions, tailored to the needs of the individual. Use a variety of modalities; drugs for pain or spasm etc., antidepressants to treat the low mood and anxiety caused by the symptoms (rather than vice versa), counter irritation and rubbing ointments to overcome allodynia. Create expectations of improvement, ('usually settles with time'). Choose which area to focus on with the patient, increasing their engagement ('so OK, let's concentrate on trying to help your sleep by working on relaxing the spasms').

Negotiate medication, ensuring that side effects are not becoming part of the problem (which can happen with analgesic headache etc.). Offer appropriate CBT, access to expert patient programmes, referring for physiotherapy and exercise if appropriate. Negotiate ways to measure the outcome the patient wants (e.g. pain scores, hours of sleep, how long they can tolerate touch etc). Ask patients to monitor these to see what works best. Indeed, encouraging them to focus on what is working can in itself help to modify the symptoms. Remember to maximise relevant medical treatment for any comorbidities ('treating the treatable').

Working on the relationship

Where there is no clear cut pathway to follow, doctors and patients can end up feeling stuck and frustrated, especially in these days of guidelines and protocols. A robust doctor – patient relationship is a key element in care. An effective relationship is signalled by the patient trusting that the doctor is caring for them as well as is possible. Box 14.3 lists some practical tips for building trust.

Box 14.3 **Practical tips for building trust**

- Collect patients from the waiting room personally, making them feel cared for
- Use your IT system to book the next appointment *with yourself* before they leave, avoiding the risk of fragmentation and 'collusion of anonymity'.
- Write to a patient after the consultation, summarising what has been said, with extra information if available, from your research, reading their old notes etc. Patients appreciate you thinking about them in between visits

---

A doctor – patient relationship built on trust enables doctors and patients to tolerate incomplete cure, or failure. When suffering is accepted and understood, doctor and patient will be better able to cope with the long-term nature of some conditions.

Although practice and use of the consultation skills in this book will help, failures will happen. Persisting in feeling one has to maintain a doctor – patient relationship when it has failed can be demoralising and unhelpful for both parties and occasionally it may be best to ask another colleague to take over, at least for a time.

Finally, MUS is a lifelong learning issue. Medical knowledge will change as will social patterns of illness. Keep practising, seek feedback from patients and colleagues, read about better ways to relate to patients and remain interested and optimistic. Time and a good doctor – patient relationship will soothe and heal many problems.

Further reading

Bub B. *Communications Skills that Heal*. Radcliffe Publishing, Oxford, 2005.

Greenhalgh T, Launer J. *Narrative Based Primary Care: A Practical Guide*. Radcliffe Publishing, Oxford, 2002.

Silverman J, Kurtz S Draper D. *Skills for Communicating with Patients*. Radcliffe Publishing, Oxford, 2005.

CHAPTER 15

Cognitive Approaches to Treatment

Vincent Deary

Department of Psychology, University of Northumbria, Newcastle, UK

OVERVIEW

- CBT can be effective for a wide range of functional symptoms
- Cognitive approaches do not aim to uncover the cause, they address perpetuating factors for symptoms
- CBT is not about 'thinking yourself better', rather it looks for logical, but counterproductive thoughts that may be acting as obstacles to a natural recovery

---

This chapter and the one that follows describe the CBT approach to medically unexplained symptoms (MUS). CBT, when delivered by specialist therapists, has been shown to be effective for many of the individual MUS syndromes and for patients with complex and multiple symptoms. A popular conception of CBT is that it is essentially a kind of positive thinking. On the contrary, CBT is about realistic, objective thinking, using reason and reality to test out beliefs.

The aim of these chapters is not to turn GPs or other generalists into CBT practitioners. Rather they aim to show how a CBT model of MUS looks in order that (a) generalists using some of the techniques in other chapters will see their parallels or origins in CBT and (b) generalists considering referring patients for CBT understand more of the treatment aims and processes.

CBT – 'it's NOT all in your mind'

When it comes to MUS, medicine and psychiatry still tend to fall back on the Freudian default. The psychoanalytic assumption is that MUS are messages from the unconscious: the person is distressed and unaware of it, but that distress will out, if necessary as physical symptoms.

People with MUS often come to CBT expecting this interpretation of their symptoms. Instead CBT seeks to build an alternative model of the condition, one in which the word psychological rarely figures. This chapter looks at CBT models, and then at some of the more common specific cognitive strategies. These should be considered in conjunction with the behavioural strategies in the next chapter.

CBT is not particularly concerned with making a diagnosis, or of considering anything – even anxiety or depression – as purely

psychological problems. Rather, a CBT therapist seeks to understand the particular interactions of body and mind – of thoughts, feelings, behaviour and physical symptoms – that an individual is experiencing, and how those interactions *maintain* their distress. In short, CBT is interested in a problem formulation, not diagnosis. Let us see how this works in practice in MUS.

Scenario 1

'David' is a 37-year-old lecturer in law, with a 1-year history of unexplained fatigue, hoarseness and loss of voice. As a result of these symptoms, he has had a lot of sick time over the past year. He is currently on summer holidays, but dreading returning to work. He has always been prone to worry and low mood, and describes himself as real perfectionist who pushes himself hard.

The current problem started about a year and a half ago, when he took up a new post, lecturing in an area of law that he didn't know very well. This triggered a lot of anxiety, and he became convinced that he was going to be 'found out' as a fraud. As result of this, he was studying this new subject for up to 16 hours a day, dropped his social life, stopped going to the gym and was sleeping badly. On top of this he was lecturing more than he ever had.

After about 6 months of this he got a throat infection and lost his voice. Initially he tried to keep going by doing everything but lecturing, but he was so exhausted that he was forced to take to bed. Two weeks later he tried to go back to work, but found his voice was unreliable and he still felt very weak. Since then it had got a little better, but his voice was still hoarse and unreliable, and he still felt exhausted and stressed.

A CBT formulation

A CBT formulation has three key parts – the three Ps. What are the *Predisposing, Precipitating* and *Perpetuating* factors of the client's distress? In Scenario 1, David has clear predisposing and precipitating characteristics (see Table 15.1). He might also have become locked in a vicious circle, where his perfectionist tendencies and his new job conspired to keep him in an activity cycle that was wearing him out – both vocally and generally. The third P, the perpetuating factors, is commonly presented as a framework of physical, emotional, cognitive and behavioral elements (see the lower part of Table 15.1). Together these three Ps make a coherent

ABC of Medically Unexplained Symptoms, First Edition.
Edited by Christopher Burton.
© 2013 John Wiley & Sons, Ltd. Published 2013 by John Wiley & Sons, Ltd.

Table 15.1 Example CBT formulation using 'the three Ps'.

Predisposing factors
Prone to distress both mental and physical (may be genetic, early life, etc.)
Perfectionist

Precipitating factors
Major transition
Prolonged period of overactivity
Prolonged period of voice use
Viral infection

***Perpetuating* factors**

Physical factors	*Cognitive factors*
Hoarseness	'I'm not good enough'
Fatigue	'I'm going to be found out'
Autonomic arousal	
Behavioural factors	*Emotional factors*
Overexertion followed by prolonged rests	Anxious
Time off work as the only way of stopping	Stressed
All energy going into work and preparation	Frustrated

narrative about why David got symptoms in the first place, and what is now keeping them going.

Developing and sharing a formulation

Remember that most patients with MUS already have multiple possible causes in mind and are looking for their clinicians to find the right one. The CBT model should include these – but instead of picking one single cause, it includes multiple factors. Developing this kind of model may be unfamiliar territory for some patients. You might say something like this:

Often there isn't one single thing that causes or keeps these kinds of symptoms going. Usually they start at a period in a persons life when they are overstretched, through work commitments, big life changes or general illness and run-downness. It sounds like in your case . . .

At this point you can illustrate this by using a framework like the one found in Table 15.1 and start to fill in the various sections of the framework. This could include some of the predisposing and precipitating factors you have identified. It is acceptable to include issues relating to personality, if the person has identified that it may be a factor :

. . . it sounds like during this time, not only were you under a lot of strain, but you were also pushing yourself quite hard to achieve a high standard, which may inadvertently have put even more strain on the system.

So that covers the first two Ps. Now introduce the third.

Again what we know from conditions like this, is that once they start, it can often be a combination of things that keep them going. I'm going to show you how this works as a vicious circle. So, you say that your voice sometimes goes, and that you get really run down. And when that happens you also feel like this . . .

Put in here, for instance, that at this point the client gets worried about losing their voice.

And the kind of thoughts that go through your head are that 'My voice is really vulnerable; if it goes again I'll lose my job'; and as a result you tend to stop using it and withdraw.

Try to highlight the connections between the factors, showing how the domains interact:

Now it sounds like this has an effect on your mood too, it gets you more down, which probably, in turn, leaves you feeling more run down and your voice weaker.

Now add more connections between physical symptoms and thoughts, feelings and behaviour. Figure 15.1 shows how cycles of thoughts, feelings and behaviour build up.

Using a formulation to introduce treatment

Building up a formulation leads naturally into a treatment rationale, a reason for working on thoughts and behaviours to change symptoms and feelings.

So, working on some of these factors might not only help with your general well being, but may also have an impact on your voice. For instance, you say that you are generally run down, so working on sorting out your sleep and activity might help you feel generally more energetic, and that may affect your voice. Also, it looks like you do push yourself quite hard sometimes, so maybe working on you going a bit easier on yourself might help you slow down a bit and feel less exhausted and stressed . . .

Of course, the patient may have other ideas, disagree, or have more to add to the picture. This process should really be a dialogue. Just keep in mind the aim of identifying the key cognitions and behaviours that are playing into the persons experience of their physical symptoms and general well-being. These are what need to change for the patient to feel better.

Engaging patients

Some patients are sceptical of this approach. Some ways to engage them in the process are suggested in Box 15.1

Box 15.1 **Engaging patients in drawing up a CBT model**

- Use physical illness analogies. Show how the vicious circle approach is used in cardiac rehabilitation or diabetes management etc
- Shift the focus from single cause to multiple factors, again illustrating how many diseases, for instance heart disease, are caused and maintained by multiple factors
- Shift the focus from cure to management. In many health complaints, like diabetes or heart disease, the focus is on management rather than cure. This does not mean that the patient is stuck with symptoms, it does however lead to more realistic therapeutic expectations, particularly in more chronic and severe MUS like CFS/ME

- Also emphasise that you do not necessarily need to know what causes a symptom to work on reducing its impact, for example the work that has been done using CBT to treat fatigue in multiple sclerosis
- Do not try and convert or change minds. Expect patients to be healthily sceptical. You are not trying to change the way they think about things; you are trying to broaden rather than challenge their illness model

Working on specific thoughts

A shared narrative about the factors involved in the onset and maintenance of their symptoms is the basis and rationale of all cognitive and behavioural interventions in MUS. In Box 15.2 we see some of the most common targets for treatment laid out in a generic MUS framework. In particular Box 15.2 includes four important specific thought areas for patients with MUS: beliefs about cause; beliefs about symptom management; beliefs about self and self-standards; and beliefs of others.

Box 15.2 **Common cognitions and behaviours in MUS**

Cognitive factors

- Beliefs about cause
- Beliefs about symptom management
- Beliefs about self and self-standards
- Beliefs of others

Behavioural factors

- Illness behaviours
- Disturbed patterns of activity, rest and sleep
- Loss of pleasurable activity
- Loss of achievement

Beliefs about cause

CBT aims to broaden patients' attributions not 'correct' them. Getting involved in a debate about cause is usually not that fruitful, whereas patients can improve substantially by learning to interpret

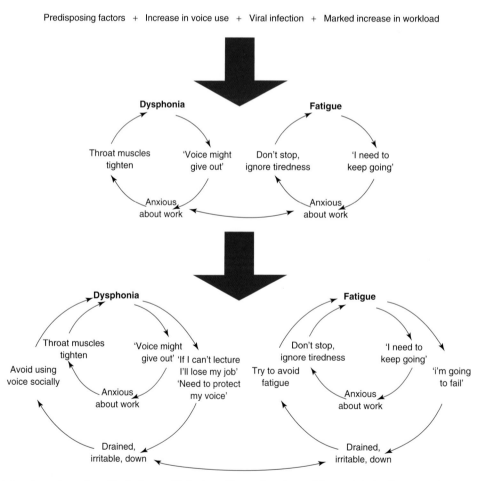

Figure 15.1 Vicious circles of symptoms, thoughts, feelings and behaviours. The predisposing and the precipitating factors on the top row lead to the top pair of circles. In turn as symptoms build up then the outer circles in the bottom pair of circles also come into play and may dominate.

and respond to their symptoms even though their causal beliefs stay unchanged.

Beliefs about symptom meaning and management

Beliefs about symptom management are a key target in the CBT approach to MUS. Two particularly common ones are that 'hurt equals harm' and the process termed catastrophisation.

Hurt equals harm

If the patient believes that symptoms are a sign of ongoing disease or 'nature's warnings', it makes sense to stop anything that provokes them. The CBT approach aims to introduce other reasons for the symptom – for instance pain sensitivity or secondary deconditioning – and add these to the vicious circles. For instance, in chronic pain, avoiding activity can lead to more weakness and sensitivity to pain, leading to more reduced activity, which can also lead to lower mood, lower self-efficacy and yet more reduced activity and pain susceptibility, and so on.

Catastrophisation

Commonly, distressed people make negative predictions, or 'crystal ball gaze'. They 'know' it will be awful, that they won't cope, will get worse and so on. They 'know' but often don't test it out.

CBT uses 'behavioural experiment' to test out these beliefs, not as a task to be endured, but an experiment to be conducted in a genuine spirit of enquiry: 'let's find out if what you believe about your symptoms is true'. This requires several components – the patient's beliefs, an agreed challenge (over which the patient needs to retain control), a shared model that links the beliefs and the challenge, and a plan for monitoring and reporting the result. Such an experiment may involve a 3 min walk for a patient with fatigue, or staying out of the toilet a little longer for a patient with IBS who catastrophises about incontinence.

CBT often uses a behavioural experiment as a form of homework between sessions, so that the patient finds out what happens when they challenge their beliefs about symptom. During behavioural experiments, symptoms usually do not improve, but are also not made worse, and self-efficacy and confidence tend to increase.

Beliefs about self and self-standards

In people with high self-standards, it is common to find particular kinds of ways of thinking about themselves and their performance, especially in those more inclined to self-criticism and perfectionism. These ways of thinking lead to beliefs like 'I am not good enough . . . and someone will find out' and 'If I don't get everything right, this is going to be a disaster'.

These beliefs play an important role in two ways. First, they may drive unhelpful behaviour and second, they may lead to stress and autonomic arousal, which in turn generates additional symptoms such as palpitations or light-headedness.

The implications of these beliefs are usually logical – if self-defeating: 'if you are not good enough, then you need to work harder even if you are exhausted'. 'If you have no time to get everything right, then you certainly have no time for fun'. A particular pattern, 'all or nothing' cognitions, is common in perfectionism: 'If I can't walk five miles like I used to, there is no point in walking at all'.

A way to gently tackle these beliefs is to enlist the patient's compassion by asking how they would respond to a best friend who was similarly driving themselves. Explore alternatives – 'if I take regular rest, I might actually perform better'; 'If I spend more time looking after myself, I might have more energy to give to my loved ones'.

Beliefs of others

People with MUS often feel dismissed by health professionals who find nothing wrong, and infer that the professionals think the condition is 'all in the mind'. This can leave them feeling misunderstood, angry or anxious that the real cause of their symptoms might have been missed. Perhaps the most important cognitions to pay attention to here are yours. Make explicit your belief in the patient's symptoms, and get along side them to work with them on the factors that may reduce the symptom's impact.

Where to start

This chapter has identified common thoughts and thought patterns that occur in patients with MUS. The best place to begin is often with something relatively simple, even if small. Pick an easy win. It will build trust and confidence in the approach. Making a small change in behaviour first – introducing a rest break after a day's work – may do more good to the patient, and your working relationship, than spending a session trying to change an illness belief. The next chapter focuses on simple behavioral strategies.

Further reading

Deary V, Chalder T, Sharpe M. The cognitive behavioural model of medically unexplained symptoms: a theoretical and empirical review. *Clin Psychol Rev* 2007;**27**:781–97.

Woolfolk RL, Allen LA. *Treating Somatization: A Cognitive Behavioral Approach*. Guilford Press, New York, 2006.

CHAPTER 16

Behavioural Approaches to Treatment

Vincent Deary

Department of Psychology, University of Northumbria, Newcastle, UK

> **OVERVIEW**
>
> - CBT works by helping patients find ways to change their behaviour and put those changes into practice
> - Behaviour change involves setting SMART (Specific, Measurable, Achievable, Realistic and Time orientated) targets and managing activity
> - Activity management includes monitoring, activity scheduling, graded changes in activity and sleep management.

Introduction

The behavioural component of a CBT approach to medically unexplained symptoms (MUS) aims to help the patient move from having their activities dictated by symptoms towards regaining some control over their life. However, the symptom-led pattern of activity is there for a reason: people avoid symptoms because symptoms are terrible. Avoiding them makes sense.

CBT, it is NOT just 'do more exercise'

As clinicians, we may know that increasing activity should help a patient's mood, pain and fatigue, but that knowledge can make us prescriptive. For the patient to gradually wrest control of their life away from their symptoms, they also need to be in control of their treatment. They need to come to a realisation that changing their behaviour makes a difference; that realisation may be hard won. The job of the clinician or therapist is to provide the patient with a plausible rationale to try doing things differently, and to offer support as the patient makes these attempts for themselves. As such, the formulation skills discussed in the previous chapter are an important preliminary to behavior change.

Know where you are going

To get better means to do better. Before beginning treatment, cognitive or behavioural, it is a good idea to get an idea of what the patient would be doing differently if they were feeling better. This

gives targets to work towards and also a clue of how to get there, step by step. Box 16.1 is an example of getting from the general aim to a particular target.

Box 16.1 **Identifying specific targets**

Therapist: *Ok, so if your pain was better, and you were generally feeling better, what would you be doing that you can't do now?*
Patient: *Well, I'd probably be socialising a lot more.*
Therapist: *What would you be doing socially?*
Patient: *I'd see my sister a lot more for a start.*
Therapist: *How often would you see her if you were feeling better?*
Patient: *Oh, probably twice a week like we used to. We used to go for coffee in our local café twice a week. I can't now, its too noisy, and I'm too worn out.*
Therapist: *Ok, so if you were feeling better, you would see you sister in your local café, twice a week. How long would you see her for?*
Patient: *Oh, we used to sit for at least an hour.*
Therapist: *And that's what you would like to do again?*
Patient: *Yes.*
Therapist: *Ok, so one of your treatment targets could be to go to the local café with your sister twice a week for an hour each time?*

This target has now moved from the general to the specific; it is now SMART : Specific, Measurable, Achievable, Realistic and Time orientated. Having established this target, the next step is to start finding steps to take towards it. For instance an intermediate goal for the patient in Box 16.1 might be seeing her sister in her own home for half an hour. The SMART goal is also a motivator. Activity towards a valued goal is more likely to be continued when things are difficult than an arbitrary goal set by the physician.

Activity management(s)

There are three types of activity management. *Activity scheduling* is useful where low mood is associated with loss of pleasure and general withdrawal or conversely where fear of failing leads to

---

ABC of Medically Unexplained Symptoms, First Edition.
Edited by Christopher Burton.
© 2013 John Wiley & Sons, Ltd. Published 2013 by John Wiley & Sons, Ltd.

overactivity. *Graded activity* is useful in pain and fatigue. *Sleep management* is used wherever there is sleep disturbance, which is a common feature of all MUS. Often, different types of activity management are used in conjunction.

Monitoring activity

The first step in all activity management is self-monitoring. When clinician and patient have identified a specific area, for instance sleep or activity, then the monitoring begins with a diary. Combined with some sleep or activity advice, this becomes the homework between sessions. In CBT it is important to emphasise that it is what people change between sessions, not what is said in sessions, that helps them get better.

Below are some of the common activity patterns in MUS that will emerge from a diary. Changing these patterns will make a difference.

Overactivity

You can spot this one because, when you go through it with the patient: you feel exhausted yourself! Overactive people sometimes devote all their energy to work. Introducing rest will be important, but equally important is variety of activity. Having fun can be as restorative as rest.

Underactivity

What is too little? When it is substantially less than they did before. If people are at home a lot, not going out much, walking little and socially withdrawn, all of these will contribute to both low mood and fatigue and experience of physical symptoms. Excessive daytime rest and/or sleep will also disturb night-time sleep.

Inconsistent or 'boom and bust' activity

This is a common pattern in MUS. It tends to follow the pattern of long stretches of activity, with little rest, followed by 'crashing out'. This may happen within a day (work all day, crash in the evening) or over several days (work all week crash at weekend). Although patients may not recognise it, this usually indicates that patients are using symptoms to dictate activity.

Loss of pleasurable activity

This can fit into any of the patterns described above, but is worth highlighting on its own. It is particularly marked in low mood where people often stop doing the things they enjoy.

Once the activity patterns become apparent, there are ways to change them. As with other things the CBT model involves presenting the client with a hypothesis – that their activity may be involved in how they feel, and that by changing their activity pattern they can change how they feel. This is a process of negotiation, and collaboration is essential.

Activity scheduling

This is useful for low mood, loss of pleasure or pleasurable activities, overworking, lack of motivation.

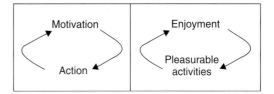

Figure 16.1 Motivation leads to action, and vice versa.

The rationale is that low mood or lack of motivation lead to stopping pleasurable activities and loss of sense of achievement. In turn this leads to low mood and lack of motivation. By deliberately 'push starting' activity again, pleasure and/or motivation will return.

Often people will say – 'I just don't have the motivation anymore, if I could only get that back, I'll start doing things again'. But the link between action and motivation is reciprocal, not one-way, as shown in Figure 16.1. When asked, most patients can think of instances where motivation has followed action rather than the other way round, or when they have enjoyed something they nearly did not do. Sometimes it helps to use analogy. A common one is starting an engine on a cold morning: you need to give it a push to start it off. Waiting for motivation to return in someone with low mood is rather like waiting for the engine to start itself.

In trying to get things started through activity scheduling, homework targets need to be SMART. So, if someone with a month's back log of work to catch up on says 'In the next week I am going to get on top of all that work stuff', it is not going to happen. Box 16.2 shows a more realistic approach to activity scheduling.

Box 16.2 **Negotiating activity scheduling targets**

Therapist: *Ok, so if you were going to start getting on top of all that work stuff, where would you start?*

Patient: *Well, I have to go through the last 2 years accounts and provide a summary report.*

Therapist: *Sounds quite daunting, what else do you have to do?*

Patient: *Well, I have a lot of unopened letters and emails to answer.*

Therapist: *Anything else?*

Patient: *I have to put together a budget for next year's planning meeting … [and so on, using open exploratory questions, you can get a fair idea of what 'all that work' means]*

Therapist: *Ok, so how realistic does it feel to you to get on top of all that stuff?*

Patient: *Well, not at all, in fact I feel exhausted just thinking about trying.*

Therapist: *Ok, so, in the next week, is there any area where you could make a start?*

Patient: *Well … I'm not sure.*

Therapist: *What would be the easiest thing to do, given that you feel quite unmotivated and overwhelmed?*

Patient: *I think I could cope with the emails.*

Therapist: *Ok, how much time could you spend on that?*

At heart the process of setting activity scheduling targets is the classic problem-solving approach, breaking big tasks down into smaller chunks. Or, as the old therapy proverb puts it, 'How do you eat an elephant? Bite by bite'.

Graded activity

This is useful for dealing with symptom-led patterns of activity.

The rationale is that physical symptoms remind us to do less and avoid difficult situations. This is a sensible short-term response. But over a long time, the less we do, the less we are able to do and when we try to do anything this leads to more physical symptoms. One way out of this vicious circle is very gradually to start doing things again, even when there are symptoms.

This process starts by looking, with the patient, at the activity diary. A common pattern in severe MUS is for the patient to be fairly inactive (either physically or socially), especially compared with how they were before they became ill. The aim of graded, or gradually increasing activity is to rebuild activity levels and confidence, so as to reduce the impact, if not the experience, of symptoms. Initially, this approach may seem counterintuitive, and the patient will need to feel the sense of it for themselves by experimenting with setting daily goals that are not determined by symptoms. The steps in graded activity are as follows.

Establish a baseline

The first step is to establish a fairly consistent routine. The aim is to set a baseline that smoothes out the peaks and troughs between and within days.

Graded increases on baseline

The second step is to make a small increase in some activity and then allow some time (5–14 days) to get used to this new level, before the next small manageable increase. It is important to recognise that during any form of graded activity, things often get worse before they get better. At some point, changes in activity will cause more symptoms and it is important to anticipate some symptom increase. It can help to think of it as the body adjusting, but as many MUS patients have catastrophic cognitions, it is valuable to plan with the patient how to interpret these symptoms as signs of change rather than of danger or damage.

Review

Any new step in graded activity needs to be reviewed at the next session. Things rarely go to plan, so adapt. Maybe they tried the walk but it really hurt. So, how about a shorter walk instead? Therapist and patient engage in a process of target setting and evaluation. Targets are increased only when the person is not feeling any worse than when they started, not when they are feeling better. Sometimes it can help to use the analogy of training to run a marathon. The first training run may be half a mile and the runner feels exhausted. By the end of the training the feeling of exhaustion may be just the same – but it takes 26 miles to bring it on.

Sleep management

Sleep management is useful for disturbed sleep for whatever reason: low mood, fatigue or worry.

The rationale is that often when we are ill our bodies get out of their usual rhythm and sleep becomes disturbed. People may

Table 16.1 Sleep management

Advice	Rationale
Get up at the same time every day	In people who are ill, their getting up time is often erratic, and dependent on what time they fell asleep This disrupts the natural sleep–wake cycle and worsens tiredness The best way to re-set this clock, is to get up at the same time every day
Go to bed around the time you normally fall asleep, or when you really feel sleepy	People who are tired often go to bed early, but do not get to sleep for hours Aim to stay up until roughly the time the person currently falls asleep
Have a good night-time routine	Stop work or vigorous exercise by early evening; no caffeine, not too much alcohol Get into pyjamas, brush teeth, have a hot bath (not necessarily in that order). These signal to the body that it is time to sleep
If you are not asleep after about half an hour, get up and do something else boring instead	Lying in bed 'trying to get to sleep' never works If they are not asleep within half an hour, advise the patient to get out of bed, do something restful, and try again when they feel sleepy
Cut-out daytime sleep	Sleeping during the day can be a hard habit to break once established. It is best to start with the idea of substituting rest, or brief napping, for deep daytime sleep Suggest setting an alarm clock for an agreed amount of time. Set an achievable initial target, then slowly decrease it at a rate the patient is comfortable with
Reducing sleep	There is good evidence that it is possible to sleep too much. Aiming for less sleep in the long run, will make patients feel less, not more tired What is needed here is a good rationale and a gradual collaborative approach, particularly as this goal seems initially quite counterintuitive
Worry time	To reduce sleep disruption from anxiety, set a time in mid-evening to think about difficulties or make lists for tomorrow If this worry comes up when they are trying to get to sleep, they remind themselves that it is in hand. The very act of getting stuff onto paper can alleviate a lot of worry

sleep more than they used to, or less, or have poorer quality sleep. Re-establishing a good sleep routine can help physical symptoms, mood and energy levels.

As always this begins by recording what is currently happening, in a sleep diary. This notes what time the patient goes to bed; what time they start trying to get to sleep; what time they fall asleep; if they wake up in the night, and for how long; what time they wake up for the last time; what time they get up. This can be used to identify patterns that might be keeping a disturbed sleep cycle going. Some of the most common ones are: a lot more time spent awake in bed than asleep, a very variable getting up time, daytime sleep, too much or too little sleep.

Working on sleep is based on a few simple strategies. The key is in negotiating SMART objectives and then applying them consistently over time. Table 16.1 describes several strategies that can be used in this process.

Summary

All of the commonly used behavioural techniques described in this chapter are there to be used flexibly rather than prescribed by rote. They are adaptable and should be modified for the individual patient. The can be, and are, used in the management of physical symptoms irrespective of cause, such as fatigue in multiple sclerosis.

Above all, it is important to keep coming back to a shared model of the problem and its treatment. The better the patient understands what they are doing, and why, the more likely they are to take over the management of their own condition, which is the ultimate goal of all good CBT interventions.

Further reading

Deary V, Chalder T, Sharpe M. The cognitive behavioural model of medically unexplained symptoms: a theoretical and empirical review. *Clin Psychol Rev* 2007;**27**:781–97.

Woolfolk RL, Allen LA. *Treating Somatization: A Cognitive Behavioral Approach*. Guilford Press, New York, 2006.

CHAPTER 17

Pharmacological Treatment

Killian A. Welch

Robert Fergusson Unit, Astley Ainslie Hospital & University of Edinburgh, Edinburgh, UK

OVERVIEW

- There is good evidence supporting the use of antidepressants in functional somatic symptoms; patients do not have to be depressed to derive benefit
- Other atypical analgesics such as gabapentin and pregabalin can also be useful
- This group of patients often tolerate drugs poorly due to a combination of sensitivity to side effects and the nocebo response

---

Introduction

This chapter will address four points: how drugs appear to work for medically unexplained symptoms (MUS); choosing which drug to use; explaining treatment; and side effects including the nocebo response.

How drugs appear to work for symptoms

When considering drug treatment for patients with MUS it can be helpful to think of five symptom groups as targets for treatment; pain; functional disturbance (e.g. other abnormalities of sensation, movement disorders, palpitations); fatigue; depression; and anxiety. Occasionally, other psychiatric diagnoses such as hypochondriasis, post-traumatic stress disorder (PTSD), psychotic illness, obsessive–compulsive disorder or even dementia may need to be considered for specific treatment.

Reducing depression or anxiety

Obviously if depression and anxiety are prominent, benefit can arise through treatment of these. However, the benefits of antidepressants and some anticonvulsants extend beyond this, although the mechanisms by which they work have been most studied for pain.

Reducing central sensitisation to pain

The brain is not only important for interpreting incoming stimuli and relating them to previous memories, but also has an important buffering effect on ascending pain signals. The descending antinociceptive system (and potentially analogous systems for other sensory stimuli) that acts as a filter or 'pain barrier' to incoming signals, may be defective in functional syndromes such as fibromyalgia and IBS. Antidepressants and anticonvulsants may act by enhancement of these descending antinociceptive effects, normalising a system that has lost some natural filters and barriers.

Altering symptom appraisal and autonomic responses

Furthermore, it is increasingly recognised that many patients with functional symptoms have an exaggerated stress response (this likely contributing to the worsening of symptoms in the context of life stressors), and have an attentional bias for unpleasant or threatening stimuli. Drugs may thus work by normalising these exaggerated endocrine and/or autonomic stress responses and by inhibition of prefrontal cortical areas that underpin 'attention' to noxious stimuli.

This physiological evidence is supported by evidence from systematic reviews that it is not necessary to be depressed to benefit from 'antidepressants'. Indeed, patients with a number of functional syndromes benefit from doses of tricyclic drugs which are sub-therapeutic for depression. People with a wide range of functional somatic symptoms appear to benefit and in many cases there is little to choose between classes except tolerability. Antidepressants with both serotonergic and noradrenergic activity (such as tricyclic antidepressants other than clomipramine, venlafaxine and duloxetine) appear to have benefit in chronic pain that is independent of any mood-elevating effects.

Choosing which drug to use

The two main classes of centrally acting drugs for managing MUS are antidepressants and anticonvulsants, however there are a few other drugs with a potential role. Table 17.1 lists a range of conditions within the MUS spectrum and summarises the options for drug treatment. Precautions in prescribing for particularly patient groups are detailed in Table 17.2

ABC of Medically Unexplained Symptoms, First Edition.
Edited by Christopher Burton.

Table 17.1 Prescribing tips for specific conditions.

Condition	Medication	Notes
Palpitations	Propranolol	Increased awareness of normal heartbeat can be helped by propranolol. It can also be helpful if other symptoms of autonomic arousal, such as exaggerated physiological tremor, are contributing to health anxiety
Tension type headache	TCAs	If not tolerated then SSRIs are likely to be a more reasonable alternative than other antidepressants
Irritable bowel syndrome	Antispasmodics e.g. mebeverine	May relieve cramping pain
	TCAs	Useful if pain and diarrhoea prominent, may worsen constipation
	SSRIs	Less useful for pain but will not worsen constipation
	SNRIs	May be good compromise if constipation and prominent pain symptoms
Chronic pelvic pain	COCP, GnRH agonist (e.g. goserelin)	Hormonal treatment may be of some benefit in those whose pain is cyclical
	Antispasmodics	If comorbid with irritable bowel syndrome
	TCAs, gabapentin	Atypical analgesia options are as for fibromyalgia (see below)
	NSAIDs	In contrast with fibromyalgia, however, NSAIDs are worth trialling in chronic pelvic pain
Fibromyalgia	TCAs	Atypical analgesic, sleep promoting and gastrointestinal effects may all be beneficial. Often benefit from doses regarded as sub-therapeutic for treatment of depression
	SNRIs	Preferable to SSRIs as greater atypical analgesic effects
	Pregabalin, gabapentin	Atypical analgesic effects and also some anxiolytic (licensed indication for pregabalin) and mood-elevating effects
Non-epileptic attacks (dissociative convulsions)	SSRIs, trazodone	If panic disorder is clearly present it should be treated aggressively, with SSRIs as first-line treatment. If it is not, or treatment is not tolerated, sedative antidepressants with anxiolytic properties (e.g. trazodone or mirtazapine can be useful)
Dissociative motor or sensory disorders	TCAs	Pain is often prominent; treating as per fibromyalgia can be helpful
Chronic fatigue syndrome	As fibromyalgia	If pain prominent treat as for fibromyalgia
		If pain not prominent SSRIs are a reasonable (non-sedating) alternative. Conversely, if insomnia prominent and TCAs not tolerated mirtazapine or trazodone worth trying. No evidence to support the use of stimulants

In these summaries it is assumed that depression and anxiety/panic disorder are not particularly prominent. If they are their treatment should be prioritised. COCP, combined oral contraceptive pill; GnRH, gonadotrophin-releasing hormone; NSAIDS, non-steroidal anti-inflammatory drugs; SNRI, Serotonin norepinephrine reuptake inhibitors; SSRI, selective serotonin reuptake inhibitors; TCA, tricyclic antidepressants.

Table 17.2 Precautions in prescribing for particular patient groups.

Medication	Precautions
SSRIs	If substantial comorbidity citalopram/escitalopram or sertraline are first choice as lower potential for drug interactions. Note recent revised dose limits of citalopram (40 mg rather than 60 mg in under 65s) with increased recognition of the potential of citalopram/escitalopram to lengthen the QTc interval (i.e. the time between the start of the Q wave and the end of the T wave corrected for heart rate as measured on an ECG)
	Bleeding risk; may want to prescribe gastroprotective drug if patient is older or on NSAIDs
	Initial increase in anxiety means often prudent to start on half dose
	Relatively safe in overdose, but need to review after initiation in case increase in suicidality
TCAs	Dangerous in overdose. Lofepramine relatively safe and (although still very dangerous) nortriptyline and imipramine less toxic than amitriptyline. Lofepramine and nortriptyline have relatively less serotonergic activity, so may not be quite as effective in pain symptoms as more dual acting TCAs.
	Avoid if recent myocardial infarction/unstable angina. Caution if co-prescribed with other QTc prolonging drugs
	Lower seizure threshold; try to avoid in epilepsy
Carbamazepine	Teratogenicity means should be avoided in women of childbearing age
Gabapentin	May worsen absence or myoclonic seizures. Evidence of safety in pregnancy lacking
Pregabalin	Evidence of safety in pregnancy lacking
Benzodiazepines	Addictive potential means best avoided in these often chronic conditions
Propranolol	Avoid in asthma. As may mask signs and symptoms of hypoglycaemia caution in diabetes. Caution in pregnancy

NSAIDS, non-steroidal anti-inflammatory drugs; SSRI, selective serotonin reuptake inhibitors; TCA, tricyclic antidepressants.

Antidepressants

There is good evidence that antidepressants are beneficial in functional somatic syndromes, with a number needed to treat for short-term improvement of approximately four. The benefit is seen in patients with and without depression. Limited data guides antidepressant choice. Meta-analyses comparing the responses of patients with headaches, fibromyalgia, and chronic pain suggest tricyclic antidepressants (TCAs) are slightly more effective than selective serotonin reuptake inhibitors (SSRI). The difference is probably greatest in patients with chronic, unexplained pain. A reasonable principle is that when pain symptoms are prominent then it makes sense to choose an agent with combined noradrenergic and serotonergic activity.

Tricyclic drugs

These are the most commonly prescribed drugs for symptoms. Most GPs are familiar with using amitritpyline for a wide range of pain syndromes including post-herpetic neuralgia. Some specialists prefer imipramine and some patients seem to tolerate nortriptyline better.

Serotonin norepinephrine reuptake inhibitors (SNRI)

Duloxetine or venlafaxine (aiming for doses above 150 mg of the latter) are reasonable choices if there are contraindications to tricyclic use. If these drugs are not tolerated, however, there is still reason to be optimistic that SSRIs can provide benefit.

Selective serotonin reuptake inhibitors (SSRIs)

SSRIs probably have a class effect. Citalopram/escitalopram and sertraline are the most commonly used in this situation.

Trazodone

The sedative, anxiolytic, non-addictive agent trazodone can be very useful if insomnia is prominent. It can also be helpful, in split doses, if anxiety is particularly prominent. Although there is a theoretical risk of serotonin syndrome and an increased risk of gastrointestinal bleeds it is generally reasonably safe combined with SSRIs.

Anticonvulsants

Anticonvulsants are useful in pain management. Pregabalin, gabapentin and carbamazepine have a clear role and lamotrigine and topiramate may also have pain-reducing effects. As many of the neurophysiological processes in pain are common to both 'explained' and 'unexplained' pain syndromes it makes sense to try these effective drugs in patients for whom pain is a major symptom, regardless of cause.

Pregabalin also has anxiolytic effects, for which it is licensed, and this property may be shared by gabapentin. Controlled trials are needed, but clinical experience does suggest that pregabalin and gabapentin have a useful role in some functional somatic syndromes.

Explaining treatment

Many patients with MUS do not regard themselves as having depression (and a good proportion are right!). Consequently, if you are prescribing a psychotropic drug you need to explain why. If the first time your patient finds you have prescribed an 'antidepressant' is when they read the information leaflet, then it is too late. Your patient will probably feel deceived, diminished or dismissed.

You may wish to explain that antidepressants are frequently used to treat symptoms such as pain and headache and are effective even if people are not depressed. Consider explaining treatment in terms of correcting physiological processes: for instance restoring the nerve pathways that act as symptom filters or barriers. When prescribing an anticonvulsant, again make it clear that this is not for epilepsy. Some clinicians find it is useful to consider the analogy of other drugs that have multiple uses, for instance aspirin being used to treat a headache or to thin the blood.

Remember that many people still think of antidepressants as addictive, you may need to counter that.

As these patients are particularly prone to side effects (see below) drugs should be started at low dose and increased gradually. A 'script' for discussing the initiation of antidepressants is suggested below. As will be clear from the discussion above this does actually reflect what we know about the actions of these drugs rather than being disingenuous.

Pain like yours often needs something as well as painkillers in order to build up pain resistance in the nerves. X is a drug we often use to do this. It started out as a treatment for depression (and if you read the leaflet in the pack it says that), but it works just as well for pain in people who don't have depression.

Reviewing and discontinuing drugs

Often, before the diagnosis became clear, a variety of unnecessary drugs have already been started. These can contribute significantly to symptom load. This is particularly apparent in patients with pain symptoms in whom opioid analgesia may result in fatigue, constipation and possibly intermittent withdrawal symptoms, while contributing little to symptom control.

There is no evidence that NSAIDs are beneficial in fibromyalgia, and these should be stopped. Up to 80% of people with non-epileptic attacks (dissociative seizures) in whom epilepsy has been excluded have been exposed to anticonvulsants. There is a comparable problem with anti-anginal drugs for patients with chest pain and normal arteries. Such prescriptions have the potential to cause considerable confusion for both doctors and patients, and in the case of non-epileptic attacks cessation of these drugs is associated with a reduction in frequency of attacks. Anticonvulsants should be stopped through a tapered reduction because of the risk of withdrawal seizures (see Table 17.3).

If you are the patient's GP, you will be well placed to review why particular drugs were started, if they had any beneficial effect, and whether there is any ongoing rationale for their use. Starting an antidepressant can be a good opportunity to down-titrate and stop unnecessary drugs. In the case of functional pain it can be explained to the patient that atypical analgesics such as antidepressants and anticonvulsants are more effective than NSAIDs or opioid analgesia for the sort of pain that they have. Starting them should enable discontinuation of the side-effect causing agents they are currently taking.

Table 17.3 How to stop anticonvulsant drugs (data from Oto *et al.* 2005).

Drug	Withdrawal protocol
Phenytoin	100 mg/week until dose is 100 mg/day, then 25 mg/week
Carbamazepine	200 mg/week until dose is 1000 mg/day, then 100 mg/week
Sodium valproate	500 mg/week until dose is 500 mg, then 200 mg/week
Vigabatrin	500 mg every 2 weeks until dose is 500 mg/day, then 500 mg alternated days for 2 weeks
Lamotrigine	100 mg/week until dose is 300 mg, 50 mg/week until dose is 50 mg, then 25 mg/week
Gabapentin	800 mg/week until dose is 1200 mg, then 400 mg/week
Topiramate	100 mg/week until dose is 200 mg, 50 mg/week until dose is 50 mg, then 25 mg/week
Levetiracetam	500 mg/week until dose is 1000 mg, then 250 mg/week
Pregabalin	200 mg/week until 200 mg, then 100 mg/week

Addiction to prescribed treatment

Detailed discussion of the relationship between chronic pain and addiction is beyond the scope of this chapter, but Box 17.1 summarises how to recognise addiction in chronic pain. Addiction requires the presence of aberrant behaviours, as physical dependence and tolerance alone are expected physiologic phenomena associated with chronic opioid or benzodiazepine treatment. Its prevalence in this population is estimated as 3–19%, above the population prevalence of substance addiction.

Box 17.1 **Recognising addiction to prescribed medication**

- Loss of control in the use of medication
- Excessive preoccupation with the medication despite adequate analgesia
- Adverse consequences associated with its use
- 'Probably more predictive' behaviours are selling prescription drugs, forging prescriptions, stealing/borrowing another's drugs, injecting oral form, prescription drugs from non-medical sources, misuse of related illicit drugs, more than two unsanctioned drug increases, and recurrent prescription loss
- 'Probably less predictive' behaviours are aggressive complaining about need for higher doses, drug hoarding, requesting specific drugs, unapproved use, similar drugs from other medical sources, unintended effects, and up to two unsanctioned dose increases

---

Side effects and the nocebo response

The placebo response is an important component of treatment efficacy. It is maximised by empathically creating plausible expectation for recovery and it applies to both 'explained' and 'unexplained' conditions. Unfortunately, there is an opposite to the placebo: the nocebo effect, which represents the expectation that treatment will be ineffective or harmful and that leads to increased reporting of side effects and discontinuation of treatment. Many factors appear to influence this, but low expectations arising from treatment with psychotropic agents for conditions patients regard as 'entirely physical' often plays some role.

This unfortunate reality is an important issue when discussing the effects and side effects of drug treatment for MUS. If side effects are played down too much and then experienced, trust and confidence is lost. If every potential side effect is discussed however, it is more likely medication will not be tolerated. A practical compromise is to discuss the most common side effects (e.g. the dry mouth and general feeling of lethargy associated with TCA initiation, increased anxiety and nausea with SSRIs). It is reasonable to emphasise that these generally improve as the body 'accommodates' to the drug and deal with it by starting at low dose and gradually increasing (say every week).

Even with these precautions individuals frequently tolerate drugs poorly, often necessitating the trial of several agents. It is reasonable to maximise the chances of identifying a tolerable drug by, for example, switching antidepressant classes after a failed trial. All other indications being equal, it is also reasonable to first try drugs which, pharmacology suggests, are likely to be better tolerated. Frequently however the breadth of effects of a particular agent is precisely the reason it is chosen. For example, despite its side effects, a TCA may be the first choice given its combination of hypnotic, analgesic and anxiolytic as well as mood-elevating effects.

Treatment of less common psychiatric disorders

There are a few other conditions, which are relatively uncommon but important to identify and treat, which may present with health concerns and MUS. These include obsessive–compulsive disorder and hypochondriasis. Diagnosis and treatment of these is generally the role of a psychiatric specialist but may include serotonergic drugs such as clomipramine or SSRIs in the higher dose range. If hypochondriacal beliefs are held with delusional intensity an antipsychotic drug may be appropriate.

Further reading

Fallon BA. Pharmacotherapy of somatoform disorders. *J Psychosom Res* 2004;**56**:455–60.

Jackson JL, O'Malley PG, Kroenke K. Antidepressants and cognitive-behavioral therapy for symptom syndromes. *CNS Spectr* 2006;**11**:212–22.

Oto M, Espie C, Pelosi A, Selkirk M, Duncan R. The safety of antiepileptic drug withdrawal in patients with non-epileptic seizures. *J Neurol Neurosurg Psychiatry* 2005;**76**:1682–5.

Spiller R, Aziz Q, Creed F, *et al.* Guidelines on the irritable bowel syndrome: mechanisms and practical management. *Gut* 2007;**56**:1770–98.

CHAPTER 18

Conclusion

Chris Burton

University of Aberdeen, Aberdeen, UK

This book did not set out to describe everything you might want to know about medically unexplained symptoms (MUS), but hopefully it has conveyed both specific information and an overall approach that is practical and useful.

It could not cover all topics and several problems have not been included. Atypical facial pain, temporomandibular joint dysfunction, idiopathic tinnitus, functional dysphonia, globus, the anal pain syndromes and bladder pain syndrome were all left out. It has also left out contentious conditions such as chronic Lyme disease, exposure syndromes (such as Gulf War syndrome) and multiple chemical sensitivity. However, as it has taken an approach of multiple causes including biological, neurophysiological and psychological factors the framework of assessment described does not depend on there being an organic or a functional cause.

For each of these additional conditions, the principles for understanding and managing these overlaps strongly with the subjects covered in the specific-symptom chapters – recognition, explanation, validation of the patient and their symptoms and action to address perpetuating factors. Indeed, the same principles can be used for disproportionate symptoms associated with disease – for instance disabling breathlessness despite good lung function in asthma.

This book can just be used as a reference point, but the techniques it describes are the starting point for the reader, to build valuable clinical skills. In order to help this, the Appendix contains a list of points for reflection and audit for each chapter. The list is designed to be copied and used as the basis for further work to add impact to each chapter. It can also act as a record of your time spent on this to be counted towards revalidation.

Patients with functional symptoms are a common feature of generalist clinical practice. Some can be difficult to treat, but almost all value the respect and the informed efforts of their clinicians. No one can explain functional symptoms completely, but with the techniques in this book, you should be able to make more sense of symptoms, both for your patients and yourself.

ABC of Medically Unexplained Symptoms, First Edition.
Edited by Christopher Burton.
© 2013 John Wiley & Sons, Ltd. Published 2013 by John Wiley & Sons, Ltd.

Suggestions for Reflection and Audit

Chris Burton

University of Aberdeen, Aberdeen, UK

Chapter	Reflection or audit
1 Introduction	How do *you* recognise patients with medically unexplained systems (MUS)? Give 10 patients with functional symptoms the Patient Health Questionnaire (PHQ15) 'to see what other symptoms they have'
2 Prevalence and impact	Look at a day's clinics. How many patients had either a transient or an established MUS? Audit 20 referrals to specialists for symptoms • How many turned out to be MUS? • How many had previously had MUS referrals?
3 Organic disease	Think about three cases where an organic diagnosis was delayed because you thought it was functional • Which systematic errors occurred? • What might you do differently?
4 Emotional disorders	How do you explain comorbid depression or anxiety to patients? What works and what does not when you try? Consider giving 10 patients with functional symptoms the Hospital Anxiety and Depression Scale (HADS) or PHQ9 + Generalised Anxiety Disorder Assessment (GAD7)
5 MUS and the GP	Audit your use of the types of normalisation. Keep a list handy for four clinics and note down which ones you use and when • In which situations might you have done things differently? • Plan a different approach for the patients you know will be coming back
6 Principles of assessment and treatment	Consider how you use time and silence in the conversation • Use a timer to see how long you let the patient keep talking at the start of the consultation. Try and lengthen it • Try listening for ideas, concerns and expectations without asking directly for a day. What did you find? Think of some patients where you find it difficult to explain what is going on • What do you think they think? • Write, rehearse and use a plausible and empowering explanation

ABC of Medically Unexplained Symptoms, First Edition.
Edited by Christopher Burton.
© 2013 John Wiley & Sons, Ltd. Published 2013 by John Wiley & Sons, Ltd.

Chapter	Reflection or audit
7–13 Specific symptoms	Pick one or more syndromes. Look for patients in your practice with them (10 for the common ones, a few for the less common) • Has anyone made an explicit diagnosis of a functional disorder? • Has anyone explained to the patient what is happening when they have symptoms? How could you do this better? • Have you supplied the patient with self-help information?
14 Consultation	Try using the 'what does it *feel* like' question in 10 different consultations and keep a log. What did it tell you? Consider arranging with a colleague or educational supervisor to video and observe some consultations? Plan to change a few things and describe what you find
15–16 CBT	How many patients with MUS have you referred for cognitive-behavioural therapy (CBT)? Where would you refer them? Write down how you explain what the aim of the CBT is? What assumptions does your explanation make?
17 Drug treatment	The next five times you prescribe an antidepressant or anticonvulsant for pain or symptoms note what you say. If you could say more, then write, rehearse and use an explanation with three more patients

Index

Note: Page references in *italics* refer to Figures; those in **bold** refer to Tables

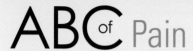

ABC of Pain

Lesley A. Colvin & Marie Fallon
Western General Hospital, Edinburgh; University of Edinburgh

Pain is a common presentation and this brand new title focuses on the pain management issues most often encountered in primary care. *ABC of Pain*:

- Covers all the chronic pain presentations in primary care right through to tertiary and palliative care and includes guidance on pain management in special groups such as pregnancy, children, the elderly and the terminally ill
- Includes new findings on the effectiveness of interventions and the progression to acute pain and appropriate pharmacological management
- Features pain assessment, epidemiology and the evidence base in a truly comprehensive reference
- Provides a global perspective with an international list of expert contributors

JUNE 2012 | 9781405176217 | 128 PAGES | £24.99/US$44.95/€32.90/AU$47.95

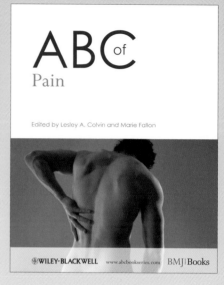

ABC of Urology

3RD EDITION

Chris Dawson & Janine Nethercliffe
Fitzwilliam Hospital, Peterborough; Edith Cavell Hospital, Peterborough

Urological conditions are common, accounting for up to one third of all surgical admissions to hospital. Outside of hospital care urological problems are a common reason for patients needing to see their GP.

- *ABC of Urology, 3rd Edition* provides a comprehensive overview of urology
- Focuses on the diagnosis and management of the most common urological conditions
- Features 4 additional chapters: improved coverage of renal and testis cancer in separate chapters and new chapters on management of haematuria, laparoscopy, trauma and new urological advances
- Ideal for GPs and trainee GPs, and is useful for junior doctors undergoing surgical training, while medical students and nurses undertaking a urological placement as part of their training programme will find this edition indispensable

MARCH 2012 | 9780470657171 | 88 PAGES | £23.99/US$37.95/€30.90/AU$47.95

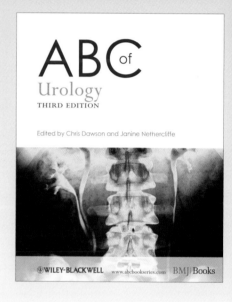

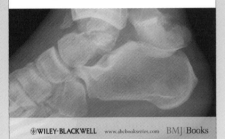

ABC of Emergency Radiology

3RD EDITION

Otto Chan
London Independent Hospital

The *ABC of Emergency Radiology, 3rd Edition* an invaluable resource for accident and emergency staff, trainee radiologists, medical students, nurses, radiographers and all medical personnel involved in the immediate care of trauma patients.

- Follows a systematic approach to assessing radiographs
- Each chapter covers a different part of the body, leading through the anatomy for ease of use
- Includes clear explanations and instructions on the appearances of radiological abnormalities with comparison to normal radiographs throughout
- Incorporates over 400 radiographs

JANUARY 2013 | 9780470670934 | 144 PAGES | £29.99/US$48.95/€38.90/AU$57.95

ABC of Resuscitation

6TH EDITION

Jasmeet Soar, Gavin D. Perkins & Jerry Nolan
Southmead Hospital, Bristol; University of Warwick, Coventry; Royal United Hospital, Bath

A practical guide to the latest resuscitation advice for the non-specialist *ABC of Resuscitation, 6th Edition*:

- Covers the core knowledge on the management of patients with cardiopulmonary arrest
- Includes the 2010 European Resuscitation Council Guidelines for Resuscitation
- Edited by specialists responsible for producing the European and UK 2010 resuscitation guidelines

DECEMBER 2012 | 9780470672594| 144 PAGES | £28.99/US$47.95/€37.90/AU$54.95

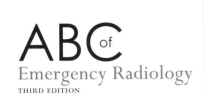

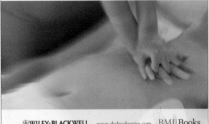

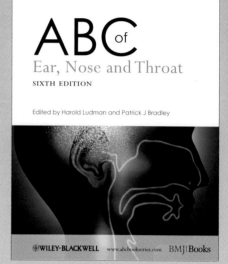
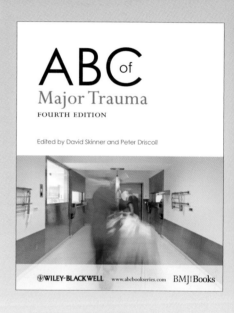

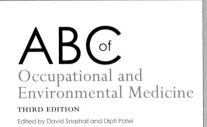

ABC of Occupational and Environmental Medicine

3RD EDITION

David Snashall & Dipti Patel

Guy's & St. Thomas' Hospital, London; Medical Advisory Service for Travellers Abroad (MASTA)

Since the publication of last edition, there have been huge changes in the world of occupational health. It has become firmly a part of international public health, and in Britain there is now a National Director for Work and Health. This fully updated new edition embraces these changes and:

- Provides comprehensive guidance on current occupational and environmental health practice and legislation
- Concentrates on the newer kinds of occupational disease, for example 'RSI', pesticide poisoning and electromagnetic radiation, where exposure and effects are difficult to understand
- Places an emphasis on work, health and well-being, and the public health benefits of work, the value of work, disabled people at work, the aging workforce, and vocational rehabilitation
- Includes chapters on the health effects of climate change and of occupational health and safety in relation to migration and terrorism

NOVEMBER 2012 | 9781444338171 | 168 PAGES | £27.99/US$44.95/€38.90/AU$52.95

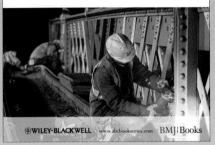

ABC of Kidney Disease

2ND EDITION

David Goldsmith, Satish Jayawardene & Penny Ackland

Guy's & St. Thomas' Hospital, London; King's College Hospital, London; Melbourne Grove Medical Practice, London

Nephrology is sometimes considered a complicated and specialized topic and the illustrative ABC format will help GPs quickly and easily assimilate the information needed. *ABC of Kidney Disease, 2nd Edition*:

- Is a practical guide to the most common renal diseases to enable non-renal health care workers to screen, identify, treat and refer renal patients appropriately and to provide the best possible care
- Covers organizational aspects of renal disease management, dialysis and transplantation
- Provides an explanatory glossary of renal terms, guidance on anaemia management and information on drug prescribing and interactions
- Has been fully revised in accordance with new guidelines

OCTOBER 2012 | 9780470672044 | 112 PAGES | £27.99/US$44.95/€35.90/AU$52.95

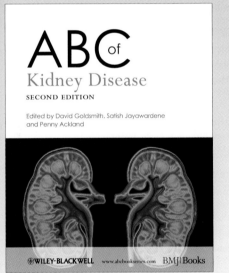

ABC of Adolescence
Russell Viner
2005 | 9780727915740 | 56 PAGES
£26.99 / US$41.95 / €34.90 / AU$52.95

ABC of Antithrombotic Therapy
Gregory Y. H. Lip & Andrew D. Blann
2003 | 9780727917713 | 67 PAGES
£26.50 / US$41.95 / €34.90 / AU$52.95

ABC of Arterial and Venous Disease, 2nd Edition
Richard Donnelly & Nick J. M. London
2009 | 9781405178891 | 120 PAGES
£31.50 / US$54.95 / €40.90 / AU$59.95

ABC of Asthma, 6th Edition
John Rees, Dipak Kanabar & Shriti Pattani
2009 | 9781405185967 | 104 PAGES
£26.99 / US$41.95 / €34.90 / AU$52.95

ABC of Burns
Shehan Hettiaratchy, Remo Papini & Peter Dziewulski
2004 | 9780727917874 | 56 PAGES
£26.50 / US$41.95 / €34.90 / AU$52.95

ABC of Child Protection, 4th Edition
Roy Meadow, Jacqueline Mok & Donna Rosenberg
2007 | 9780727918178 | 120 PAGES
£35.50 / US$59.95 / €45.90 / AU$67.95

ABC of Clinical Electrocardiography, 2nd Edition
Francis Morris, William J. Brady & John Camm
2008 | 9781405170642 | 112 PAGES
£34.50 / US$57.95 / €44.90 / AU$67.95

ABC of Clinical Genetics, 3rd Edition
Helen M. Kingston
2002 | 9780727916273 | 120 PAGES
£34.50 / US$57.95 / €44.90 / AU$67.95

ABC of Clinical Haematology, 3rd Edition
Drew Provan
2007 | 9781405153539 | 112 PAGES
£34.50 / US$59.95 / €44.90 / AU$67.95

ABC of Clinical Leadership
Tim Swanwick & Judy McKimm
2010 | 9781405198172 | 88 PAGES
£20.95 / US$32.95 / €26.90 / AU$39.95

ABC of Complementary Medicine, 2nd Edition
Catherine Zollman, Andrew J. Vickers & Janet Richardson
2008 | 9781405136570 | 64 PAGES
£28.95 / US$47.95 / €37.90 / AU$54.95

ABC of COPD, 2nd Edition
Graeme P. Currie
2010 | 9781444333886 | 88 PAGES
£23.95 / US$37.95 / €30.90 / AU$47.95

ABC of Dermatology, 5th Edition
Paul K. Buxton & Rachael Morris-Jones
2009 | 9781405170659 | 224 PAGES
£34.50 / US$58.95 / €44.90 / AU$67.95

ABC of Diabetes, 6th Edition
Tim Holt & Sudhesh Kumar
2007 | 9781405177849 | 112 PAGES
£31.50 / US$52.95 / €40.90 / AU$59.95

ABC of Eating Disorders
Jane Morris
2008 | 9780727918437 | 80 PAGES
£26.50 / US$41.95 / €34.90 / AU$52.95

ABC of Emergency Differential Diagnosis
Francis Morris & Alan Fletcher
2009 | 9781405170635 | 96 PAGES
£31.50 / US$55.95 / €40.90 / AU$59.95

ABC of Geriatric Medicine
Nicola Cooper, Kirsty Forrest & Graham Mulley
2009 | 9781405169424 | 88 PAGES
£26.50 / US$44.95 / €34.90 / AU$52.95

ABC of Headache
Anne MacGregor & Alison Frith
2008 | 9781405170666 | 88 PAGES
£23.95 / US$41.95 / €30.90 / AU$47.95

ABC of Heart Failure, 2nd Edition
Russell C. Davis, Michael K. Davis & Gregory Y. H. Lip
2006 | 9780727916440 | 72 PAGES
£26.50 / US$41.95 / €34.90 / AU$52.95

ABC of Imaging in Trauma
Leonard J. King & David C. Wherry
2008 | 9781405183321 | 144 PAGES
£31.50 / US$50.95 / €40.90 / AU$59.95

ABC of Interventional Cardiology, 2nd Edition
Ever D. Grech
2010 | 9781405170673 | 120 PAGES
£25.95 / US$40.95 / €33.90 / AU$49.95

ABC of Learning and Teaching in Medicine, 2nd Edition
Peter Cantillon & Diana Wood
2009 | 9781405185974 | 96 PAGES
£22.99 / US$35.95 / €29.90 / AU$44.95

ABC of Liver, Pancreas and Gall Bladder
Ian Beckingham
1905 | 9780727915313 | 64 PAGES
£24.95 / US$39.95 / €32.90 / AU$47.95

ABC of Lung Cancer
Ian Hunt, Martin M. Muers & Tom Treasure
2009 | 9781405146524 | 64 PAGES
£25.95 / US$41.95 / €33.90 / AU$49.95

ABC of Medical Law
Lorraine Corfield, Ingrid Granne & William Latimer-Sayer
2009 | 9781405176286 | 64 PAGES
£24.95 / US$39.95 / €32.90 / AU$47.95

ABC of Mental Health, 2nd Edition
Teifion Davies & Tom Craig
2009 | 9780727916396 | 128 PAGES
£32.50 / US$52.95 / €41.90 / AU$62.95

ABC of Obesity
Naveed Sattar & Mike Lean
2007 | 9781405136747 | 64 PAGES
£24.99 / US$39.99 / €32.90 / AU$47.95

ABC of One to Seven, 5th Edition
Bernard Valman
2009 | 9781405181051 | 168 PAGES
£32.50 / US$52.95 / €41.90 / AU$62.95

ABC of Palliative Care, 2nd Edition
Marie Fallon & Geoffrey Hanks
2006 | 9781405130790 | 96 PAGES
£30.50 / US$52.95 / €39.90 / AU$57.95

ABC of Patient Safety
John Sandars & Gary Cook
2007 | 9781405156929 | 64 PAGES
£28.50 / US$46.99 / €36.90 / AU$54.95

ABC of Practical Procedures
Tim Nutbeam & Ron Daniels
2009 | 9781405185950 | 144 PAGES
£31.50 / US$50.95 / €40.90 / AU$59.95

ABC of Preterm Birth
William McGuire & Peter Fowlie
2005 | 9780727917638 | 56 PAGES
£26.50 / US$41.95 / €34.90 / AU$52.95

ABC of Psychological Medicine
Richard Mayou, Michael Sharpe & Alan Carson
2003 | 9780727915566 | 72 PAGES
£26.99 / US$41.95 / €34.90 / AU$52.95

ABC of Rheumatology, 4th Edition
Ade Adebajo
2009 | 9781405170680 | 192 PAGES
£31.95 / US$50.95 / €41.90 / AU$62.95

ABC of Sepsis
Ron Daniels & Tim Nutbeam
2009 | 9781405181945 | 104 PAGES
£31.50 / US$52.95 / €40.90 / AU$59.95

ABC of Sexual Health, 2nd Edition
John Tomlinson
2004 | 9780727917591 | 96 PAGES
£31.50 / US$52.95 / €40.90 / AU$59.95

ABC of Skin Cancer
Sajjad Rajpar & Jerry Marsden
2008 | 9781405162197 | 80 PAGES
£26.50 / US$47.95 / €34.90 / AU$52.95

ABC of Spinal Disorders
Andrew Clarke, Alwyn Jones & Michael O'Malley
2009 | 9781405170697 | 72 PAGES
£24.95 / US$39.95 / €32.90 / AU$47.95

ABC of Sports and Exercise Medicine, 3rd Edition
Gregory Whyte, Mark Harries & Clyde Williams
2005 | 9780727918130 | 136 PAGES
£34.95 / US$62.95 / €44.90 / AU$67.95

ABC of Subfertility
Peter Braude & Alison Taylor
2005 | 9780727915344 | 64 PAGES
£24.95 / US$39.95 / €32.90 / AU$47.95

ABC of the First Year, 6th Edition
Bernard Valman & Roslyn Thomas
2009 | 9781405180375 | 136 PAGES
£31.50 / US$55.95 / €40.90 / AU$59.95

ABC of the Upper Gastrointestinal Tract
Robert Logan, Adam Harris & J. J. Misiewicz
2002 | 9780727912664 | 54 PAGES
£26.50 / US$41.95 / €34.90 / AU$52.95

ABC of Transfusion, 4th Edition
Marcela Contreras
2009 | 9781405156462 | 128 PAGES
£31.50 / US$55.95 / €40.90 / AU$59.95

ABC of Tubes, Drains, Lines and Frames
Adam Brooks, Peter F. Mahoney & Brian Rowlands
2008 | 9781405160148 | 88 PAGES
£26.50 / US$41.95 / €34.90 / AU$52.95